Midlife Matters

Katie Taylor

Midlife Matters

Feel empowered and confident every step of the way

CONTENTS

PRAISE FOR
MIDLIFE MATTERS

"A best friend's guide to midlife."

Andrea McLean, broadcast journalist, author, and coach

....

"A wonderfully helpful handbook for all midlife women, packed with highly relevant, thoughtful, and practical information and advice. There are lots of purely 'menopause' books, but this one adds so much more."

Liz Earle MBE, author, broadcast journalist, and brand founder

....

"Katie is a midlife powerhouse, that friend in your group who has the answers to anything and everything and has now written all of that down! Calling on multiple experts, she has used her knowledge to help all of us."

Dr Philippa Kaye, doctor, author, journalist, and broadcaster

....

"Start here for a warm and informative introduction to the world of midlife. Katie Taylor has assembled an array of advisors – from gynaecology, oncology, and neurology to fitness, finance, and family counselling – to guide women through the challenges of this period in their lives."

Avrum Bluming MD and Carol Tavris PhD, authors of Oestrogen Matters

....

"The perfect companion for any 40-plus woman who needs guidance through all aspects of midlife."

Dr Naomi Potter, menopause specialist, doctor, and author

....

"If midlife has knocked you sideways, this brilliant book will get you back on track. This rich and relatable guide is informed with leading experts in all areas of the midlife journey and the voices of countless women who needed to be seen, heard, and helped to revolutionize this next chapter."

Rachel Schofield, career coach, author, and former BBC News journalist

....

"This book is a bible for every midlife woman. Through bravely shared stories and a wealth of knowledge gained from specialists during her work in the midlife space, Katie helps us all to believe that this is the best chapter yet."

Rosie Nixon, author, broadcaster, and coach

....

"This is the ultimate guide to navigating midlife and menopause."

Professor Guy Leschziner PHD FRCP, Professor of Neurology

....

"Katie's drive and determination to help and educate midlife women has always been at the core of her purpose. This book is the real deal."

Michelle Griffith Robinson OLY, olympian, life coach, and motivational speaker

....

"Katie is one of the original pioneers of the menopause movement. This book contains a wealth of information and inspiration for every midlife woman who wants to craft a healthier and happier life after 40."

Nicki Williams, nutritional therapist, podcast host, and author

....

"Books like this are invaluable resources which help cheerlead and support women who can so often feel undervalued, unconfident, and unsure of how to embrace their next chapter."

Tamsen Fadal, author, journalist, broadcaster, and menopause advocate

....

"*Midlife Matters* is an essential guide for anyone navigating midlife, blending relatable storytelling with expert insights. This beautifully written book is a must-read, offering invaluable wisdom and heartfelt stories that make it the perfect gift to yourself or someone you love."

Ruby Hammer MBE, internationally acclaimed makeup artist and TV personality

....

"Katie is one of the most respected menopause campaigners in the UK. Her platform, The Latte Lounge, supports, educates, and signposts women, and this book is a wonderful extension of her expertise, humour, and understanding of the subject."

Alice Smellie, journalist and author

....

"In this book you will find a treasure trove of information, contributed by specialists in their field, that should be available to every woman in midlife. This invaluable guide will educate, inform, and empower readers to make truly informed choices."

Diane Danzebrink, author and founder of Menopause Support

....

"*Midlife Matters* should be essential reading, not only for all midlife women but also their partners, families, and wider society. With each section written by a leading specialist in their field, this book empowers women to confidently take control of their individual health as they navigate their way through the menopause maze."

Professor Nick Panay, Consultant Gynaecologist and President of the International Menopause Society

....

Introduction

Why do we need a book about midlife? Simply put, midlife presents women with a unique set of challenges. We are often referred to as the "sandwich generation", with those of us who have children combining parenting responsibilities with caring for ageing parents as well as managing the other relationships in our lives. Along with running a home and balancing work commitments, at a time when we are starting to experience a raft of mental and physical changes and challenges, it's no wonder that our own health and wellbeing ends up at the bottom of the priority list.

This stage of our lives comes without a manual, and so figuring out how to navigate this next chapter can feel daunting, isolating, and confusing. It soon becomes clear why many women liken these midlife years to living inside a pressure cooker. This is also why, according to the Office for National Statistics, thousands of women leave the workforce at the peak of their careers, and the highest rates of both divorce and suicide in women occur in midlife.

My own experiences of midlife are what inspired me to share my journey, first through a social media platform and website and then in this book. I was 43 when I began to struggle with low mood.

My usually outgoing and capable persona was slowly replaced with diminished energy, brain fog, and anxiety. As a mum of four, I put it down to the challenges of juggling a family, home, and career. For the next few years I struggled with insomnia along with a whole host of unrelenting symptoms, from heart palpitations and painful joints to crying spells and poor concentration. My periods had also become shorter and heavier, and I had gained a lot of weight.

My doctor said I was probably stressed and depressed, and suggested I take time off or give up working altogether. I was given antidepressants, but they didn't make things any better, they just made me numb; I tried going to the gym and eating more healthily, but neither helped; I was sent to a heart specialist for my palpitations, who ruled out a heart condition; to a neurologist, who ruled out early-onset dementia; I saw a rheumatologist for my joint pains. I went back and forth to several different doctors and specialists to investigate all of the various symptoms I was suffering from.

It was ultimately my father, a leading breast cancer specialist, Professor Michael Baum, who suspected that all of my symptoms were hormone-related and arranged for me to see a gynaecologist who specialized in the menopause. After an initial consultation and blood test, the doctor explained that my oestrogen levels were "on the floor", and that all of these seemingly unrelated symptoms were actually due to perimenopause (a word that I'd never even heard before). They suggested that I start on HRT (hormone replacement therapy) immediately.

On the night of my diagnosis I came home and cried with relief that I wasn't going mad and there was in fact an explanation for everything I'd been feeling. But I also felt really, really angry that so many doctors had not recognized these symptoms and I had wasted four years of precious life not really living. Within a couple of months of using HRT, I was starting to feel like my old self again. My husband commented that he felt like he'd got his wife back, and my kids their mum.

I decided there and then to start a Facebook group and website, The Latte Lounge, aimed at women over 40, so that I could share my experiences and help those who might have been in the same place as me. But I didn't want it to just be about menopause. I'd become more aware of the numerous pressures, challenges, and changes facing women in midlife, and I was determined that this should be a forum where all of these different issues could be discussed.

I put together a medical advisory team and a panel of health and wellbeing experts to support women with advice and evidence-based articles, not only about perimenopause and menopause, but also addressing all areas of midlife health and wellbeing. We talk about everything from healthy eating and hormones to fitness and finance, from the challenges around juggling work to looking after ourselves while also caring for our children, partners, and ageing family members.

The Latte Lounge is a place where women find it safe to confide in each other. Knowing that you are part of a group of like-minded women, many of whom have either been in your shoes or are currently wearing them, is not only helpful and reassuring, but in some cases it can save jobs, lives, and marriages, too. And now that wisdom and so much more is here in these pages.

I also know that access to good-quality healthcare, support, and information is not always easily available to many women, so this book aims to offer as much evidence-based, unbiased, up-to-date information as possible, from many of the world's leading experts. Here, you will find advice from more than 40 renowned psychologists, doctors, professors, dermatologists, dieticians, athletes, lawyers, and other high-profile health, wellbeing, style, and beauty experts.

Think of this as your midlife handbook: it will arm you all with the information you're looking for, in straightforward, jargon-free language, so that you can feel empowered to take on the challenges – and reap the rewards – of this exciting new life stage.

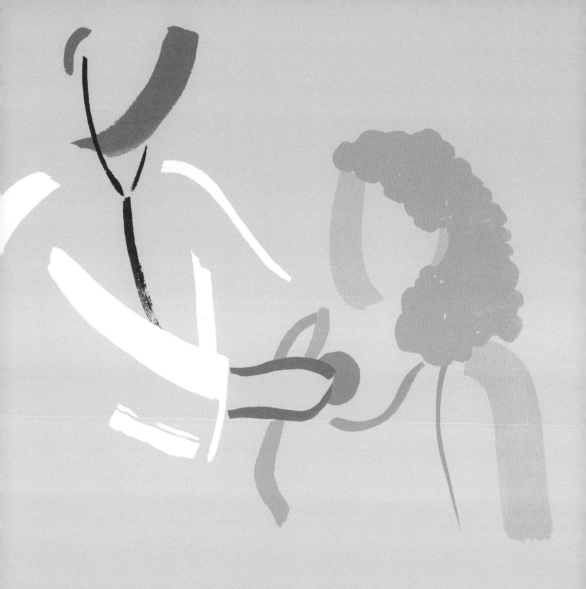

HEALTH

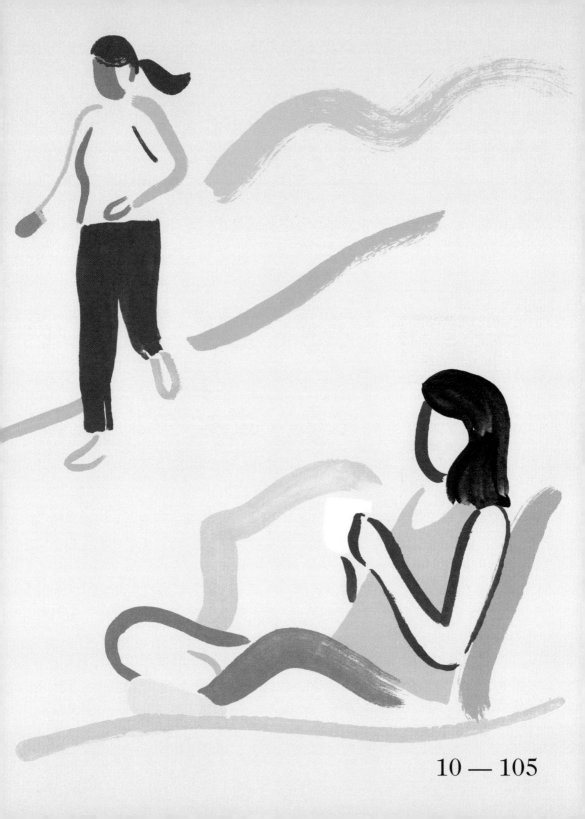

10 — 105

Menopause

Many of us find ourselves entering our 40s feeling bewildered that some things seem out of kilter and our once reliable hormonal cycle is no longer playing ball. Due to a lack of education about this life stage and a lot of fearmongering, I struggled for so long with my own menopause journey, and many women across the globe continue to do so. This chapter aims to help you understand what happens to our hormones as we age, and the impact of these fluctuating hormones on our health and wellbeing.

UNDERSTANDING THE MENOPAUSE

Do you remember learning anything about menopause at school? Had you ever heard anyone mention the word perimenopause before? No, me neither. The only thing I knew was that it was something that happened to grey-haired old ladies who were plump around the middle, red in the face, and fanned themselves a lot. So why would I have any idea of what was to come?

At school we are taught a little about the menstrual cycle, how a baby is made, and how not to get pregnant, but it was usually a rushed module to save blushes. And that's where our education on the female reproductive and fertility journey usually ended. We were certainly never told that the definition of menopause is a day and a year since your last period, or that perimenopause is the time leading up to menopause (lasting anywhere from 4–10 years), when a whole host of seemingly unrelated symptoms may start to appear. And hard as it may be to believe, there has also been little focus on menopause education in the curriculum of medical students, too.

When I came across Diane Danzebrink through The Latte Lounge, I was shocked to hear how her experience of the menopause took her to an even darker place than my own did, and why it eventually led her to start a national campaign.

In July 2012 I had a total hysterectomy, including the removal of both of my ovaries, as it was suspected that I had ovarian cancer. Prior to my surgery I received no information about the potential impacts or symptoms of being plunged into surgical menopause (see. p.18) or how to manage them.

A few months after surgery my mental health deteriorated. I became increasingly anxious and lost my confidence. I started to experience panic attacks, and I spent most nights lying awake desperate for sleep.

Work became completely impossible as I just couldn't concentrate. I left the house less and less and was reluctant to see friends, answer the phone, or open post, which I was convinced would only contain bad news.

The world felt dark and scary, and having woken after another horrendous night I remember thinking, I can't do this anymore. Later that day I came within moments of taking my own life.

Having told my husband what I had almost done he immediately contacted our doctor's practice. The doctor I saw that night explained that I was experiencing severe menopause symptoms due to the drastic reduction of oestrogen caused by the removal of my ovaries. She explained the benefits and risks of body identical HRT and she assured me it was what I needed.

The HRT patch she prescribed made a difference very quickly. The world no longer felt like such a dark, scary place – but relief soon turned to anger. Looking back at what I had almost done made me wonder how many other women were suffering due to a lack of the right information and support. I promised that if I ever felt like myself again, I would make damn sure I did something to change the menopause landscape for the future.

I founded Menopause Support in 2015, a purpose-over-profit organization, offering education, information, guidance, and support. In October 2018, I launched the national #MakeMenopauseMatter campaign in Westminster, lobbying for menopause training for all doctors and medical students to be made mandatory, for menopause guidance and support to be available in every workplace, menopause included in the new RSE curriculum in schools, and a public health campaign for menopause. Over 200,000 signed the petition. Menopause is now on the school curriculum in England and medical students now learn about menopause, but there is much work still to do.

DIANE DANZEBRINK, FOUNDER OF MENOPAUSE SUPPORT

Diane's experience is sadly not an isolated case; there are altogether too many women whose symptoms have led them to despair. This is why I am determined to ensure that these stories become a thing of the past, and have been campaigning with Diane for years, alongside many other grass roots campaigners, high-profile supporters, and menopause specialists to ensure that, in Diane's words, "We will be the generation to make menopause matter." With the right education and support, this natural stage of our lives can be both empowering and rewarding. It's important to note here that anyone assigned female at birth (AFAB) can be impacted by the menopause, so while we refer to women throughout the book, many issues can also affect trans men.

We will be the generation to make menopause matter.

—

Q & A
Professor Nick Panay, Consultant Gynaecologist,
President of the International Menopause Society

What is menopause?

In the simplest terms, it means that you have gone for 12 full months without a period. Menopause affects all women, and it can also affect transgender and non-binary people too.

What are the four stages?

1. PRE-MENOPAUSE
This is the phase of life when you have no symptoms and your periods will be generally regular. The ovaries are fully functioning in healthy women, and hormone production is ongoing. For many this phase begins in the early teens and continues through until the early to mid-40s, but for some it can end a lot earlier.

2. PERIMENOPAUSE
The months and years leading up to menopause, which on average in the UK will begin around the age of 45, although it can start earlier or later. During this time periods will become infrequent and irregular, and you may experience symptoms such as hot flushes, night sweats, and low mood.

3. MENOPAUSE
This is actually a single point in time – the one day directly after 12 months since your last period. In the UK and the US, the average age that a woman reaches menopause is 51 years old. This is lower in some Asian countries, such as India, which is around 47 years of age.[1]

4. POSTMENOPAUSE
This is the period of time after your diagnosis of menopause. It doesn't necessarily mean that your menopausal symptoms will have ended, but it does mean that your periods will have stopped.

What causes the menopause transition?

It is part of the natural ageing process when our body's hormone production begins to change. The exception to this is if surgery, chemotherapy, or other medical intervention causes an early (before 45) or premature (before 40) menopause.

What happens to the body and mind during this transition?

The cells in our body thrive on oestrogen, progesterone, and testosterone, so when these levels fluctuate and fall during the perimenopause and menopause it can trigger many different changes in our bodies. Some women will experience psychological symptoms, others physical symptoms, and many will experience both (see right).

How can we recognize symptoms of perimenopause and menopause?

Different women will have different symptoms, and some will have few or none. The classic symptoms of menopause are hot flushes and sweats, vaginal dryness, and pain during sexual intercourse. Some symptoms are directly due to menopause, and some are also due to the ageing process. This is why it's recommended to use a symptom checklist so that you can review the symptoms together with your healthcare provider to work out an individualized plan. You do not need to experience all of these symptoms to be in perimenopause or menopause.

What is GSM? (Genitourinary Syndrome of Menopause)

GSM is commonly known as vulvovaginal atrophy (VVA) postmenopausally, and more than 50% of women suffer from it. As oestrogen levels decline, the pelvic area can be adversely affected, leading to vaginal dryness, pain during intercourse, urinary urgency, urinary tract infections, and even incontinence (see pp.64–71). The symptoms can be embarrassing and feel taboo to discuss with your healthcare

provider, but it's so important that you do so that you can be treated effectively and safely.

Symptom Checker

PHYSICAL

- Allergies
- Bloating
- Body odour
- Bone fractures
- Breast soreness
- Brittle nails
- Burning mouth
- Decrease in libido (sex drive)
- Dental and gum problems
- Dry, itchy skin
- Dizziness
- Joint pain
- Hair loss
- Headaches
- Hot flushes
- Irregular periods
- Muscle tension and restless legs
- Nausea and digestive issues
- Night sweats
- Palpitations
- Tingling extremities
- Tired or low energy
- Urinary symptoms
- Vaginal dryness
- Weight gain

MENTAL

- Anxiety and loss of confidence
- Brain fog and poor memory
- Depression or low mood
- Difficulty concentrating
- Difficulty sleeping and disrupted sleep
- Irritability
- Mood swings
- Panic attacks and panic disorders

What are premature and early menopause?

For around 1–4% of women, menopause will happen much earlier and occur under the age of 40; this premature menopause is medically defined as "premature ovarian insufficiency". Early menopause occurs between the ages of 40 and 44.

What if they are left untreated?

If they are not treated with hormones (either HRT or the contraceptive pill), premature and early menopause can significantly increase the risk of brittle bone disease (osteoporosis), heart disease, dementia, and even Parkinson's disease.

What are surgical and medical menopause?

Sometimes menopause can happen more suddenly and before the natural ageing process. This can be due to surgery, for example if the ovaries are removed in a hysterectomy, or it can be because ovaries are damaged by medical treatments such as chemotherapy or radiotherapy to treat cancer and blood disorders. The sudden loss of hormones can have a profound effect on wellbeing and quality of life, and it is imperative that a good plan is made to ensure that adequate support is provided, and hormones are replaced (unless this is contraindicated).

How long does the menopause transition last?

The length of each stage of the menopause transition varies for each woman. The average length of perimenopause is approximately 4–5 years, but some women may be in this transition phase for many more years. Symptoms can last for 7–8 years on average.

How long do symptoms persist postmenopause?

The duration of symptoms in the postmenopause stage is variable; symptoms do usually continue from peri- to postmenopause before they eventually improve. In 5–10% of women the symptoms can continue indefinitely.

When should I see a doctor about my symptoms?

If your symptoms are troubling you, please do not suffer in silence – make an appointment to talk to your doctor.

If you are over 45, take a copy of your symptom checker and your own notes about your symptoms to your appointment. If you are under 45, it is particularly important to report your symptoms; in this age group hormone therapy will not only alleviate suffering but will also provide protection against osteoporosis and heart disease.

How is menopause diagnosed?

Your doctor should be able to diagnose if you are in perimenopause or menopause based on your symptoms (including how often you have periods) as well as your age. A blood test may be offered if you are under 45, and definitely if you are younger than 40, in order to confirm the diagnosis.

How should women prepare for their doctors' appointments?

Preparation is key as often doctors' appointments are short, so summarize how you are feeling and what you need help with beforehand, and be clear about the questions you want answered. It may also be a good idea to take your partner or a close friend or relative with you, because if you are suffering with brain fog or extreme exhaustion you can often forget or feel overwhelmed by all the information that is discussed.

What are the options for those who are suffering with symptoms?

There are many options to consider when it comes to treatment, and there is no one-size-fits-all. Before considering hormonal treatments (see pp.20–23) or pharmacological alternatives it is important that any treatment strategy is underpinned by optimizing your lifestyle choices. When it comes to using supplements,

always take a "food-first" approach and try to get as many of your nutrients as possible from a balanced, healthy diet (see pp.110–119). If you do decide to use supplements, it's important to choose wisely as there is little regulation over the supplement industry.

You can read in much more detail about lifestyle choices and self-care in the Wellbeing chapter of this book (see pp.106–166, and check the summary box below); I would recommend you do, because if you have mild symptoms, lifestyle choices alone can make a huge difference and may be all that you require.

If you have tried these approaches and you are still suffering with your symptoms then it's important to have an informed conversation with your healthcare provider about HRT and/or other therapies and pharmaceutical options.

Lifestyle Changes

- Minimize alcohol consumption
- Avoid smoking
- Increase exercise and activity levels
- Adopt a healthy diet
- Get a good night's sleep
- Manage your stress levels

HORMONE REPLACEMENT THERAPY (HRT)

The decision about whether or not to take HRT can be a big one, regardless of the benefits that you will read about here. You may have concerns about its safety, whether it's an "unnatural" thing to do, or whether there are any unwanted side effects.

Doctors and researchers now agree that HRT is a safe option for most women in menopause to replace the hormones that are lost. But there is sometimes misleading information in the media about HRT, much due to a now de-bunked 2002 study[2] that claimed HRT may increase the risk of breast cancer. A large and growing bank of evidence demonstrates that it is safe for most women, but always discuss your options with a menopause specialist. It is so important that every patient makes an informed joint decision with their own medical team, because there are many factors involved in assessing personal risk, including genetics, family history, and lifestyle aspects such as alcohol consumption, diet, and exercise.

When I interviewed BBC Radio broadcaster and journalist Kirsty Lang for The Latte Lounge, she told me that she was diagnosed with breast cancer at the age of 53. She had been on HRT for four years previously to manage her menopause symptoms, and her surgeon suggested she stop taking it as there was a slightly raised risk of breast cancer returning if she continued. Kirsty stopped at once, but her resulting symptoms were so severe that she eventually made the decision to resume HRT after assessing that it was worth the risk in order to enjoy a better quality of life. Kirsty advises women to "Have the courage to make an informed decision yourself about what's right for you. I felt that my life was too miserable off HRT, and that not taking it wasn't doing me any good."

Doctors and researchers now agree that HRT is a safe option for most women.

—

Q & A
Professor Nick Panay, Consultant Gynaecologist,
President of the International Menopause Society

What is the role of HRT?

HRT replaces the hormones that are lost as women go through menopause. There is no way to reverse the decrease in hormone production in our bodies, so HRT is the only way to replace them.

What are the benefits?

HRT is designed to restore the natural pre-menopausal hormonal environment, which will ease many symptoms caused because of the low hormone levels, especially hot flushes, night sweats, and vaginal dryness. Some other potential benefits of HRT are bone and heart protection. Testosterone can usually be added if low libido is a persistent problem.

Is HRT safe?

HRT is a safe option for most women in menopause. Much of the older evidence that unfortunately led to concerns was disproven because of serious limitations in the studies. We now have many different types of more natural hormone therapy, which can be used to truly individualize treatment, minimizing risks and maximizing benefits. Some women may experience minor adverse effects when they first start

HRT, including breast tenderness, bloating, and breakthrough bleeding.

The risks of thrombosis and stroke is minimized with lower doses of tablets or by using patches, gels, or sprays. The risk of breast cancer is minimized by using more natural "body identical/body similar" types of progesterone. Side effects of testosterone can include excess hair growth and spots, but are improved by reducing the dosage or stopping treatment.

How long will it take for HRT to help my symptoms?

It can take a few weeks before you feel the benefits, and up to three months to experience the full effects. It may also take your body time to get used to HRT. Some women may need to tweak the type of HRT being used and the dose during the first few months to alleviate any side effects or bleeding problems.

How long can I stay on HRT?

This will vary depending on your individual circumstances. The good news is that there is no set length of time. Some women choose to take it for just a few years to offset the worst symptoms of menopause, and find they then have no more symptoms after they stop. It's best to review your decision each year with your doctor.

What options are there for women who have had a hysterectomy?

Most can have HRT. Usually oestrogen-only is prescribed, unless it is thought there may be residual endometriosis. Testosterone is given if there's an impact on sexual desire that does not respond to conventional HRT.

It is vitally important that if women have had a surgical menopause (see p.18) they receive appropriate HRT so that one problem is not replaced by another.

What about for women who are in premature menopause?

It is important to get individualized hormone therapy right for everyone, but particularly for women in premature menopause as they're going to be in menopause for so many years of their lives. Younger women generally require higher doses of hormone therapy to control their symptoms, at least until the average age of menopause (51 years).

Is HRT a contraceptive too?

No. HRT should not be regarded as being contraceptive unless the combination being used includes a progestogen-releasing intrauterine device (hormone-releasing coil). This combination can be useful for women in the perimenopause requiring both HRT and contraception. If there is any doubt about your menopausal status, use contraception while taking HRT and continue using it until the age of 55.

Can I take HRT if I have had cancer?

The side effects of cancer treatment can trigger menopausal symptoms, and for these women treatment options may appear limited because there aren't many evidence-based drugs available currently that are totally safe for cancer patients. However, benefits can often outweigh the risks, so it is important to have a joint informed risk discussion with a specialist. HRT should still be an option for women with persistent distressing symptoms, but initially lifestyle, dietary, and exercise options should be discussed.

Pharmacological alternatives should also be considered: some have a reasonably good evidence base for effectiveness, including antidepressants like venlafaxine or bladder drugs like oxybutynin.

Cognitive behavioural therapy (CBT) has been proven to help many manage their symptoms. The new neurokinin receptor antagonist medications are now available for treating hot flushes and sweats and may also help with sleep and mood. The first one has recently been licensed in the UK.

Mental Health

Within The Latte Lounge community, there are so many conversations with women who say they are struggling with life, feeling "burnt out" and suffering with anxiety and/or depression, many of them forced to quit their jobs because they just can't cope. But no matter what our mental health has looked like to date, it's important that we give ourselves the time and space to deal with these concerns now in order to protect our current and future mental health.

TAKING STOCK AND SEEKING HELP

I'm sure we all know someone who has struggled with their mental health over the years, or perhaps you have personally suffered due to any number of reasons. Often this is because of the midlife pressures placed upon women, be that caring for the various needs of our children and/or ageing parents, dealing with stresses like financial concerns and work pressures, or perhaps coping with a breakdown in a relationship. But quite often it's also to do with our hormones plummeting; symptoms of the perimenopause and menopause can be misdiagnosed as anxiety and depression (as was the case for me). Sometimes women may have gone through life with undiagnosed conditions that are now being "unmasked", such as dyslexia, ADHD (Attention Deficit Hyperactivity Disorder), OCD (Obsessive Compulsive Disorder), and ASD (Autism Spectrum Disorder), and which make coping with the day-to-day demands of life that much harder.

Before you can assess your current mental health, it's helpful to be able to recognize what good mental health looks like. While we all have bad days and mental health can look different for everyone, there are key signifiers that healthcare professionals are trained to watch out for.

When you are in good mental health you generally feel empowered and able to manage what life throws at you, in control of your thoughts and emotions, and like you can face challenges and take advantage of opportunities. On the flip side, poor mental health can manifest as living under a dark cloud, where you feel there is no hope and everything is pointless. You might feel disconnected, and powerless to make changes.

Many of us have become so used to operating below par that we have forgotten how it feels to be functioning at an optimum level. It can be hard to know who we should be going to for help, and what the journey of care should look like. This chapter seeks to address these concerns, beginning by looking at the mental health issues faced by women in midlife, followed by a more in-depth examination of how menopause impacts on anxiety, depression, and neurodivergence, and an introduction to psychological therapies that are available.

Women may have gone through life with undiagnosed conditions that are now being "unmasked".

Keep an open mind and discuss all the symptoms you have experienced rather than looking to get confirmation of a particular diagnosis or seeking a specific treatment.

—

Q & A
Dr Sophie Behrman, NHS Consultant Psychiatrist

Why do so many midlife women suffer with their mental health?

Studies show women to be at risk of first episodes of mental illness in their 40s and 50s, and are at highest risk of suicide aged 45–49.[3]

There are a number of reasons why women's mental health may deteriorate in midlife: it might be that social pressures become more intense, with caring responsibilities for generations above and below, increased responsibilities at work, and pressures due to society's negative reaction towards ageing (and in particular towards older women).

We know that entering the perimenopause can cause psychological symptoms like low mood, anxiety, and brain fog as hormones decline. For some women this may lead to a new diagnosis of a mental disorder, or an exacerbation of a pre-existing condition. The most common symptoms that women present with in midlife are low mood and/or anxiety (see pp.27–34).

Why are some women affected by depression more than others?

As with all mental health problems, the development of depression is likely due to many factors: our genetics, early life experiences, and personality type can have

an impact on how we perceive and interact with the world. Further life experiences, lifestyle factors, and other mental and physical health problems can make it more or less likely that someone develops a particular mental disorder.

Where can women go for help if they suspect they may have a mental health disorder?

If you have concerns about your mental health I would advise seeing your doctor. Keep an open mind and discuss all the symptoms you have experienced rather than looking to get confirmation of a particular diagnosis or seeking a specific treatment. Your doctor will assess you and recommend a treatment plan: this may include lifestyle changes, medication, or talking therapy, often a combination of some or all of these. Most women with mental health problems will be able to be treated by their doctor and not need to see a psychiatrist. In the NHS, patients are referred to a secondary care mental health team only when their presentation is complex and/or first-line treatment options have not helped.

When we are suffering with mental health problems, it is natural to turn to the internet to make sense of our experiences as there is a wealth of information and personal accounts, which may help us understand what is going on. However, the diagnosis of mental health problems is complex, and it is particularly hard to judge our own experiences when we are in the midst of them, so googling your symptoms is not always helpful.

What are the treatment options for poor mental health?

This depends a lot on the underlying difficulties, and doctors look at both a specific diagnosis (which may lead to a particular treatment, such as medication) and also the complex factors behind the presentation. For example, if financial problems are a strong contributory factor, we would advise specialist support in managing this alongside treatment for the mental disorder.

For treatment of specific disorders we follow protocols established in National Institute for Health and Care Excellence (NICE) guidelines.[4] Things become more complicated when the perimenopause or menopause may be contributing to mental health problems (see pp.12–23). There is some evidence that HRT in conjunction with the standard medical treatments for mental disorders may be more effective than psychiatric treatment alone.[5]

Problems rarely occur in isolation, and for most people with a mental health problem in midlife there will be a combination of predisposing and precipitating factors in its development.

Is medication enough?

This is a very individual decision and depends on what the patient has tried before and what they would like to consider for this episode of illness. I would rarely just prescribe medication without thinking about possibilities of self-help strategies, talking therapy, or other psychosocial interventions.

Cognitive Behavioural Therapy (CBT, see p.40) has a good evidence base for a number of psychological and physical health problems including low mood/depression, anxiety, pain, and symptoms of the perimenopause. A psychologist will assess you if you are referred for CBT and decide with you if it is the right therapy for you.

Do women of colour experience more intense symptoms of menopause, including anxiety and depression?

We know that in the UK the experience of menopause is different across various ethnic groups,[6] with women of South

Asian and Afro-Caribbean origin tending to have a lower age of menopause than Caucasian women. We do not understand the physiological reasons behind this, but there are also differences in how the menopause is viewed and experienced in different cultures and in where women can turn for support with their symptoms.

The relationship between ethnicity and mental illness is also complex and there is evidence that people from BAME communities are at a higher risk of developing severe mental disorders such as schizophrenia.[7] There are still inequalities in the provision of services and experiences of mental health care for BAME patients,[8] and addressing these injustices is a priority for UK mental health care.

How does the perimenopause impact on neurodiversity?

Neurodiversity means that the brain is wired differently to a "neurotypical" brain and responds in a different way to neurotransmitters (chemical signalling molecules in the brain). Whereas the goal with a mental disorder is treatment to lead to recovery, with neurodiversity we look to manage the environment and the symptoms in order to optimize the patient's experiences rather than to work towards a "recovery".

Symptoms experienced in perimenopause may mimic ADHD symptoms, for example brain fog, poor concentration, and irritability, or patients with underlying ADHD may find it gets worse during perimenopause. There is also evidence that other forms of neurodiversity, such as Autism Spectrum Conditions can be "unmasked" during perimenopause.

If you do suspect you have ADHD, doctors in the UK will do a screening questionnaire and, if the score is significant, they will refer you to an ADHD clinic for assessment, which will include a full psychiatric history and examination to look for symptoms of ADHD and to exclude other possible explanations. (See pp.35–37 for more information about ADHD in women.)

ANXIETY AND DEPRESSION

Anxiety and depression during midlife are two of the
most debilitating and commonly reported symptoms of
perimenopause and menopause. In a survey The Latte
Lounge carried out with fertility company Fertifa in 2021,
which asked a group of 500 women to share the most
troubling symptoms that they had experienced during
perimenopause and menopause, 84% of respondents said
anxiety and depression.

For many women, myself included, this is often the first
time these symptoms have appeared; for others they have
suffered for many years. But trying to decipher what the
cause may be and what we can do to feel better can be
one of the most frustrating parts of getting the correct
diagnosis. This was certainly the case for Tessa, a nursery
school head teacher, who shares her story below.

*I started suffering from severe anxiety and depression in my mid-40s. I tried
everything to deal with it – a mixture of anti-anxiety meds and antidepressants,
upping doses and switching brands – and over a five-year period saw
numerous doctors, psychiatrists, healers, therapists, and reflexologists, but
nothing helped. It got so bad that I could barely function, I stopped eating,
stayed in bed all day, and getting dressed was a huge effort. The anxiety was
so bad that I couldn't even go into a shop to buy milk. I became a shadow of
the woman I once was and was forced to give up my much-loved job.*

TESSA, 52

Many women, like Tessa, will be offered anti-anxiety or antidepressant medication to try and relieve their symptoms. For some these can be hugely beneficial, but for others, especially those whose symptoms are due to perimenopause or menopause, they may merely mask the problem. For these women it could be that HRT and/or making lifestyle changes is the more appropriate treatment (see pp.19–23). It's so important to get the right diagnosis and treatment rather than trying to put up with symptoms that can have a massive impact on your ability to function at home and in the workplace.

Depression is also very common in the perimenopause and early menopause, and its cause is often complex. One survey reported that 45–68% of perimenopausal women present with depressive symptoms, and in up to 30% of women, symptoms can be severe enough to be classified as depressive disorder.[9] Data from an American SWAN study (Study of Women's Health Across the Nation)[10] concluded that other risk factors for depression during the perimenopause and menopause include: a past history of depression; stressful life events; a past history of anxiety disorder; genetic predisposition; and poor social circumstances such as financial difficulties or unemployment.

If you are suffering from anxiety and/or depression I want you to know you are not alone: so many women do, and I personally had always prided myself on being a really upbeat person until I hit perimenopause. I felt ashamed, and almost like I was being ungrateful for all the good things I did have. Once it was explained to me that my anxiety and depression were symptoms relating to my plummeting hormone levels, I felt enormous relief. So please don't be afraid or embarrassed to mention it to your doctor, because the sooner you do, the sooner you can get the appropriate support, advice, and treatment options to help you start feeling better.

Q & A
Dr Wendy Molefi-Youri, Doctor and BMS accredited
Menopause Specialist, Founder of Vital Wellness Clinic

What is anxiety?

Anxiety is a state of hypervigilance. Your body produces adrenaline and cortisol to prepare you for a fight or flight response, and these hormones are churning around in preparation. Anxiety has a spectrum, and you can feel anything from slightly uneasy to totally overwhelmed or have a full-blown panic attack.

Symptoms of Anxiety

- Feeling on edge
- Being uneasy, irritable, and restless
- Feeling sick or experiencing an unsettled tummy that you can't explain
- Having a dry mouth

Why do anxiety and depression affect us in midlife?

Menopause has a direct effect on brain chemistry as fluctuating or declining oestrogen levels lead to an increased risk of mood disorders such as anxiety and depression. Most of us will experience anxiety at some time in our lives, but in perimenopause and menopause it can suddenly come out of nowhere. For some women it might be circumstantial, but for a vast majority it is most often due to the falling hormone levels.

When oestrogen levels go down, cortisol levels go up: cortisol is a stress hormone and higher levels will increase feelings of anxiety. We have an abundance of oestrogen receptors in the amygdala, hippocampus, and hypothalamus – the parts of the brain that are responsible for mood regulation. Oestrogen plays a significant role in mood regulation in a number of ways; it appears to protect brain cells and enhances the function of serotonin and dopamine, which are chemical messengers involved in the regulation of mood.

What reasons might there be besides hormonal effects on our mood?

The physical effects of the perimenopause and menopause can also indirectly affect our mental health. For example, night sweats can disturb sleep, so you wake up feeling tired and struggle to concentrate. This can make you feel less effective and reduce confidence and self-esteem, leading to low mood, anxiety, and depression. Hot flushes can also cause stress and anxiety, for example if you're worried about having a hot flush during a work meeting or presentation. During perimenopause you may also find yourself feeling on edge about how your periods will affect your day-to-day routine as they become less predictable or heavier.

Quite often at this time in our lives we are also taking on new responsibilities such as caring for our ageing parents and juggling the pressures of bringing up our children, and we may also be reinventing our careers or starting a new chapter in our personal lives.

All of this can also severely impact on your sleep and your ability to function, so it's little wonder that anxiety can take hold for so many women during midlife.

Why are some of us more affected by anxiety and depression than others?

We are all different and our genetics do play a role. Those who struggle at this time may have also done so postnatally or during menstruation, so past medical history and also underlying mental health issues can mean a predisposition, but lifestyle factors such as work stresses, loneliness, or adjusting to an empty nest can contribute.

For some women from religious or ethnic minority communities there are also cultural differences in how they deal with anxiety and depression: it can be embarrassing or taboo to discuss these symptoms or the impact on their mental health openly, and some communities don't even have a word for the menopause. This can lead to a vicious circle where these women suffer in silence without the support that they need.

What are the treatment options for anxiety and depression?

There are some very simple steps we can all take to help improve our own mental health without a visit to the doctor. Give yourself the time and space to take stock of your current lifestyle and see if there are any changes you can make to help you feel better (see over the page). If you've managed to address most of the lifestyle changes that could be responsible for your anxiety or depressive mood and they're not resolving it, there are over-the-counter treatments (OTC) and medical options that you can explore with your doctor too. When it comes to OTC treatments, supplements like red clover,

Symptoms of Depression

- Low mood
- Loss of pleasure
- Negative thoughts
- Low self-esteem
- Poor concentration
- Low energy
- Sleep and appetite changes

black cohosh, and St John's Wort can be helpful, but these can interact with other prescribed medicines so always check with your healthcare professional.

What about medication?

Psychological symptoms are complex, and as such a thorough assessment is crucial. If it is clear that the anxiety or depression is perimenopause or menopause related, first-line treatment would be HRT, as recommended by NICE, the statutory body that publishes guidelines in the UK. For those who do not want to take or cannot take HRT, talking therapies such as Cognitive Behavioural Therapy (CBT) have been shown to be beneficial.

The role of antidepressant medications such as SSRIs (Selective Serotonin Reuptake Inhibitors), which work by boosting levels of serotonin (the "happy hormone") in the brain, is not very clear; however, in my clinical experience some women do notice improvement in their symptoms after taking them.

Lifestyle Changes

- **Diet:** it's important to start to see food as medicine and make a conscious effort to eat things that will boost your wellbeing. If you don't know where to begin, talk to a nutritional advisor who can help to start you on the right path (see pp.108–119).

- **Exercise:** this boosts endorphins, clears your mind, and improves sleep quality – which in itself is nourishing. It doesn't have to be strenuous, a half hour brisk walk or some yoga is quite often more than sufficient (see pp.120–131).

- **Drinking:** it's essential to really try and reduce your alcohol intake. Although at first it seems to have a calming effect, alcohol can actually exacerbate anxiety and depression quite quickly.

- **Talking therapies:** take a proactive approach to your mental health. Talking therapies like CBT have been shown to be incredibly beneficial in helping you to develop coping strategies (see pp.38–41).

- **Mindfulness:** try a mindfulness practice such as meditation. If this isn't something you've tried before, there are apps that you can download to provide some structure and help you to get started (see pp.140–143 and p.248).

LIVING WITH ADHD

Our society is built around a "neurotypical" brain, so navigating this world with an ADHD brain can be overwhelming. People who are neurodiverse, such as those with ADHD, often have to adapt their environments to make life more manageable. In recent years, various research has uncovered how ADHD has been historically underdiagnosed in women, having been focused more on fidgety schoolboys. But for women living with ADHD, the perimenopause and menopause can potentially be even more of a turbulent time, with symptoms being exacerbated by fluctuating hormones.

Q & A
Dr Emma Ping, Doctor specializing in the menopause and ADHD

What is ADHD?

ADHD stands for Attention Deficit Hyperactivity Disorder. We think that it is caused by an abnormality in neurotransmitters such as dopamine and noradrenaline and changes in the structure and function of the brain, so some areas are smaller. It has only been approximately within the last ten years that women have been recognized as potentially having an ADHD brain, so many have previously been misdiagnosed or undiagnosed. There are officially three types that ADHD is grouped into:

- Inattentiveness
- Hyperactivity
- Impulsivity

An individual may be diagnosed with the predominantly inattentive type, the predominantly hyperactive and impulsive type, or a combined type of ADHD.

How does ADHD affect women?

ADHD affects the part of the brain concerned with emotional regulation. Emotional dysregulation is still a very new area, but it's definitely there and is very debilitating. Examples include: flying off the handle with anger, rage, tearfulness and despair, extremes of emotions beyond what would be the normally accepted boundaries, and impulsivity. Women with ADHD can therefore feel more vulnerable. Over time ADHD can detrimentally affect self-esteem, with many women feeling shame and inadequacy because they think that they can't do things in the way that society expects: they might find that their house is messy; they may interrupt people when they're talking; communication in relationships can be difficult.

ADHD Symptoms in Women

- Disorganization and overwhelm
- Anxiety and depression
- Hyperactivity: this can be subtle such as fidgeting, or internalized as restlessness
- Feelings of underachievement
- Time blindness

Why do so many women go undiagnosed for so long?

Young girls are more likely to have the inattentive type of ADHD, so their behaviour is less likely to disrupt the classroom and they are often trying hard to mask and do what is expected of them. The lack of disruption means their ADHD is less likely to be identified, and in the education and medical worlds, the focus of ADHD diagnosis has historically been on boys and men.

How do hormones influence ADHD?

Our current understanding is that an ADHD brain is low in dopamine, involved in executive function and emotional regulation, and oestrogen influences neurotransmitters like dopamine and serotonin. A sufficient oestrogen supply to the brain seems to help maximize the availability of dopamine, so is particularly important when an ADHD brain is already low in dopamine.

Sex hormones such as oestrogen also directly affect functions of the brain including cognition, memory, and emotion. Addressing oestrogen supply to an ADHD brain can therefore lead to improved executive function, memory, decision making, and emotional regulation.

What happens during perimenopause?

The fluctuation and decline in oestrogen can lead to ADHD-like symptoms such as brain fog and emotional difficulties in a neurotypical brain. For an ADHD woman, low oestrogen and dopamine can lead to overwhelm and difficulty functioning. There's an overlap between the symptoms of the low oestrogen and low dopamine, and so it can be challenging trying to identify what symptoms are ADHD and what are caused by perimenopause.

How can you get a diagnosis of ADHD?

Find a trained clinician. It doesn't have to be a psychiatrist, but they need to have had specialist training in ADHD assessment and diagnosis. It's a good idea to do some preparation before an ADHD assessment. There are self-tests you can find online, including the ASRS V 1.1.[11] Look for female-specific self-assessments on their website.

Some people worry about being labelled, but a diagnosis can open the door to understanding yourself better. After a diagnosis some people initially feel elation, validation, and relief, followed by grief for what could have been and anger about the past. After a diagnosis of ADHD, I would advise giving yourself a lot of compassion and seek help and support to move forward.

Treatment Options

- **Medication:** ADHD responds to stimulants (such as methylphenidate, commonly known by the brand name Ritalin), which can come in short-acting or long-acting forms, and non-stimulants (such as atomoxetine).
- **Hormone therapy:** if fluctuating female hormones are influencing your symptoms, seek help with this (see p.20–23).
- **Lifestyle changes:** exercise, meditation, and mindfulness have been shown to help (see pp.120–131, pp.140–143).
- **Rest:** Allowing time for relaxation and prioritizing sleep is important (see pp.132–139 as sleep problems are common in ADHD.
- **Talking therapies:** CBT for ADHD can be especially helpful (see p.40).

I'm 43 and have spent my life always 'on the go', but have also always been very disorganized, anxious, forgetful, and overwhelmed, and my mood swings – which have been a staple throughout my life – over the last few years have been off the scale, with rage like I've never experienced. One of my friends said she thinks I may have ADHD, but my doctor keeps brushing it off as 'just a bit hormonal'. I have no real support.

PATRICIA, 43

PSYCHOLOGICAL THERAPIES

When women go through perimenopause and
menopause, symptoms of anxiety and depression can
be very severe for some, hence the 45–49 reported
age of peak suicide in women (see p.27). Some women
turn to professionals for help; others might adopt
unhealthy coping mechanisms such as drinking, smoking,
or disordered eating, and over time go on to develop
addictions or behaviours that make things even worse.
It's no wonder that in midlife the cracks begin to appear,
leaving too many of us feeling flat and burnt out. How
can we get to the bottom of what's causing our angst and
begin to redress any ingrained and damaging habits?

Q & A
David Gittelson, Psychotherapist and Founder of the Green Door Practice

What are some of the common coping mechanisms that you see?

We learn from a young age that
when things are painful, difficult, or
uncomfortable we want to put as much
distance between us and the source of
the pain as fast as we can. This is what
promotes and perpetuates the cycle of
avoidance of these difficult feelings.

If we never address this pain, which
can often fester for months or years, then
the problem never gets dealt with and
the mind and body throw up various
symptoms, such as feeling anxious, as a
warning sign or call out for help. These
symptoms are uncomfortable, and so
quite often we use coping mechanisms
to mask or dull them. Unfortunately,
some of these coping mechanisms (such
as smoking, drinking, eating disorders,
gambling, or shopping) can become
addictive and exacerbate the original
issues and symptoms further.

It doesn't really matter if the original
issue that had led to you using these
coping mechanisms was biological or
circumstantial (such as being in an abusive

relationship – for organizations that can offer help in situations such as this, see p.249), because either way the symptoms and emotions you are experiencing or trying to bury are painful. What does matter is that the sooner the original issue can be acknowledged and addressed, the quicker you can start to heal.

When should women seek help?

Unfortunately women don't tend to reach out for help early enough, instead waiting until they are totally "burnt out". Many midlife women might express feeling overwhelmed, anxious, depressed, stressed, and like they are no longer coping. It is the doctor's job to decipher if there is an underlying medical or hormonal cause (such as symptoms of the menopause, see p.17), and if so to decide if they need further tests and/or a prescription. Or, if they feel it's more likely there are circumstantial reasons, they might first recommend talking to someone, which is often when the journey to a talking therapy starts.

What are talking therapies?

These are psychological treatments for emotional and mental health problems. They can help you find time to address whatever issues you are struggling with or are concerned about in a safe, impartial, and confidential space, supported by a trained therapist. No matter what the issue is, the job of any therapist is to identify what's going on and relay that to a patient in a way that is palatable, then find a creative way to address what it is that they're not dealing with.

The most important element is the relationship between the patient/client and the therapist. If a client feels they cannot trust the therapist, cannot be honest and open with them, doesn't feel that the therapist "gets" them, and doesn't want to spend an hour talking with them, it won't work. I often say to my clients, "Therapists are like shoes, they don't all work for all occasions. Find the right fit for you."

Are talking therapies enough?

For some women, talking therapies alone will be enough, whereas for others a combination of medication and talking therapies may be more effective. You can usually access these support services through a referral from your own health care professional, or refer yourself privately without involving your doctor.

There are many different types of therapy, but ultimately all of them are coming at the same problem from a different angle, and quite often what happens is that many people start mixing and matching, to find an approach that works for them. One approach, which borrows various elements from a range of therapeutic approaches, is called Integrative Therapy.

What are some of the different types of talking therapies?

COGNITIVE BEHAVIOURAL THERAPY

The aim of CBT is to change the way we think and act in order to manage problems. It is based on the idea that our behaviour, thoughts, and feelings are closely linked and influence each other. Unhelpful feelings and thoughts can lead to unhelpful behaviours, which can turn into a vicious cycle of experiencing even more negative thoughts. CBT teaches us to recognize these patterns and deal with problems in a different way.

CBT is practical and often challenges clients to engage directly with the problem in ways that just talking doesn't. It is also focused, ensuring direct engagement with the issue to be addressed.

COUNSELLING

This involves a trained therapist listening to you and helping you find ways to deal with emotional issues. Sometimes the term "counselling" is used to refer to talking therapies in general, but counselling is also a type of therapy in its own right.

PSYCHOANALYSIS

This a very stereotypical and classic type of therapy. The therapist generally says very little, and the work focuses on unconscious feelings and often centres on the patient's childhood.

PSYCHODYNAMIC THERAPY

This borrows from the ideas of psychoanalysis but is more discursive. It also focuses strongly on what is not being said (the unconscious ideas), what is not being thought of, and what is not being connected with. By making unconscious ideas more conscious it's hoped that the patient will feel less burdened.

RELATIONAL SCHOOL

The emphasis here is on the relationship between the client and therapist rather than what is actually said, and using that as an agent for change.

Traditional psychotherapy focused on making the unconscious mind of the patient conscious through the interpretations of the therapist, but the approach here is less about what is unconscious in the mind of the patient and more about what can be achieved in the life of the patient through a nurturing and honest relationship with the therapist.

BODY THERAPY

This is more focused on the body, breathing, and/or touch. Therapists often refer to the "psyche and the soma" (the mind and the body); somatic therapy deals with the body, whereas traditional talking therapy focuses on the mind.

These days there is a growing acknowledgement that the two should not be viewed in quite such distinct terms, and therapies such as Breath Work, Dance Therapy, Massage Therapy, Yoga, and

Pilates acknowledge that there is a link between emotional wellbeing and physical movement.

When would more specialist support be appropriate?

I often work with people who are showing signs of being addicted to a substance or struggling with addictive behaviours. When it comes to substances (like alcohol and drugs) rather than behaviours, then talking therapies alone may not be enough in helping people to detox. If I identify this issue I would usually recommend that my client seeks a specialist, either as an outpatient or inpatient, for medical care because their health may be at risk.

It is important to note that often the symptoms of depression and anxiety can be due to many other biological medical reasons, such as an illness or symptoms of the menopause, which is why it's important to establish early on if more specialist support is needed first.

What if someone is already receiving medical treatment and has a diagnosis?

Regardless of whether someone has been prescribed medication, once they find themselves in my clinic or the clinic of any good therapist, the main feature of the work we do is that we take a step back and look at what is actually going on without trying to label it, and then to try and think about what's at the root of it. I don't officially diagnose people, but for those that have already been given a diagnosis, I try to help them reassess it.

Understanding the specifics of "disorders" is not particularly helpful to the individual, but what is useful is to understand that many people get diagnosed with one or more mental health disorders or conditions/labels, and the truth is that they all display overlapping symptoms, which are incredibly similar. It's the job of the therapist to try to work out what is the fundamental cause of those symptoms, rather than simply being in a rush to label them.

CBT teaches us to recognize these patterns and deal with problems in a different way.

Brain Health

Although our mental health and our brain health are related, they are not the same thing. While mental health is concerned with mood, feelings, thoughts, and behaviours, brain health focuses on having optimal cognitive, emotional, and social functioning, free from damage or disease. There are many variables that can influence the health of the brain, from genetics to our environment and everything in between, but, as with any other organ in our body, it's vitally important we look after it now to prevent problems as we age.

BRAIN FOG

When you think about problems with the brain, perhaps the most common conditions that come to mind will be dementia and Alzheimer's disease, or maybe headaches and migraines. But there's a less obvious issue that commonly affects women in midlife: brain fog.

Before my early 40s, I had never once given the health of my brain a minute's thought. The only time brain health had ever come up in conversation was when my good friend's father tragically developed dementia, but other than that it felt like nothing for me to be concerned about. That was until I hit the age of 43, and for the first time in my life developed what can only be described as brain fog. One incident, during the Monday morning school run, made me realize I needed to get some help.

I was convinced I had driven the car to school but couldn't find it anywhere and was in a state of blind panic. Other parents offered to help me look, but couldn't resist teasing that I'd forget my head one day. Although I'd laugh with them, I was embarrassed and secretly concerned that something was very wrong with my brain. Another mum eventually drove me home, only to discover that the car was still sitting on my driveway.

Over time, my lack of memory became more and more frustrating and embarrassing: if it wasn't the car, it was my keys; if it wasn't the keys, it was my phone. And if it wasn't my possessions, it would be things like walking into a room and not remembering why I'd gone in there.

I had always been so capable, never forgetting things, always managing to juggle the responsibilities of my home and work life well. But now I felt like I was constantly walking around in a fog.

My work was severely impacted. Some days I'd stare at a budget spreadsheet and it would be like reading a different language. I couldn't concentrate at all, and felt that any minute my boss would realize I was a fraud, incapable of doing my job. I was terrified that this might be the start of early-onset dementia. It would be years before I discovered that I was far from alone in feeling this way. Sarah, a partner in a law firm, described her own experience of brain fog to me, over the page.

The only way I can describe it is as a feeling of disconnect, that I was going through the motions, but my brain was disconnected. It felt as though someone had pulled out the plug and the contents of my brain had poured down the sink, like in a Tom & Jerry cartoon.

Years of valuable knowledge gained at law school and throughout my subsequent years as a lawyer had just disappeared. I felt incapacitated: how could I continue to do my job when my clients were relying on me to remember key facts and represent them in court? I was convinced I was developing Alzheimer's.

My doctors could find nothing wrong, and eventually I was diagnosed with burnout and depression and written off from work for six months. Things deteriorated and I became paranoid to the point where I was convinced that, as well as dementia, I must have a brain tumour that was causing the fog. I had to give up my career, which had a huge impact on us financially and put massive pressure on my relationship with my partner.

SARAH, 48

Just like Sarah, my experience of brain fog also led me to give up my much-loved job, something that is not uncommon among women in midlife. In fact, results from a Latte Lounge survey with reproductive healthcare specialists Fertifa showed that 42% of women polled considered leaving their jobs due to menopause symptoms, with 87% experiencing brain fog and difficulty concentrating.[12]

We know that the pressures of midlife and effects of fluctuating hormones can have a huge impact on our bodies, but what many of us don't realize is that it can impact our brain health too; this lack of knowledge causes many of us to worry that symptoms such as brain fog could be a sign of something more sinister.

42% of women polled considered leaving their jobs due to menopause symptoms, with 87% experiencing brain fog and difficulty concentrating.

—

Q & A
Dr Philippa Kaye, Doctor and Author

What is brain fog?

Brain fog is a very poorly understood
condition that has come to the fore in
recent years. This is not only because
of menopause, but also because a large
number of people suffering from long
Covid are complaining of very similar
cognitive problems to women in
perimenopause. So it's important to try and
understand the difference between these
complaints and those that you would
expect to present in early-onset dementia
(see pp.48–49).

Brain fog isn't really a medical term in
the same way that we might use terms
like "urinary tract infection", nor even a
symptom, such as palpitations. Rather, it is
used to describe a collection of symptoms.
Some women often say their head feels as
though it is full of cotton wool, and worry
that they frequently forget where they've
put things, or can't remember people's
names or what something is called,
perhaps starting a sentence and losing
track midway through.

This happens to everyone occasionally,
but with brain fog the symptoms are
more frequent and affect daily life. The
symptoms can impact on mood, and
people are often anxious that something
serious is going on with their brain.

Cause & Effect

SYMPTOMS

- Being mentally tired or exhausted
- Difficulties with memory
- Experiencing confusion
- "Losing" words
- Finding it hard to concentrate

POSSIBLE CAUSES

- Sleep deprivation
- Stress
- Viral infections (such as Covid)
- Hormonal changes
- Mental health issues
- Fibromyalgia
- Chronic fatigue syndrome
- Chemotherapy

Why does brain fog happen?

Many people experience brain fog at some
point in their lives, perhaps after a baby is
born or around the menopause, but for
most it improves with time. Hormonal
changes during the perimenopause and
menopause can cause brain fog due to
declining oestrogen and fatigue.

Oestrogen has many roles in the brain, such as improving brain connectivity and increasing blood flow. It also affects the production of serotonin, a chemical involved in mood and executive function, which is a combination of concentration, memory, and thinking. So when oestrogen levels fall, there are changes in the brain that can result in symptoms.

How might brain fog impact our lives?

The impact will vary depending on its severity, and also from person to person, but it can be severe, leading people to give up, reduce, or change their work, and it can seriously affect relationships and self-confidence. If the brain fog is related to insomnia (see p.133–139), or low mood due to the menopause (see p.17), then treating these, for example with HRT, may help to improve symptoms. However brain fog doesn't tend to last forever, and generally gets better with time.

How do we know if it's more serious?

If you notice a change and are concerned, then get checked out. The perimenopause and menopause have lots of symptoms and it is easy to assume that everything must automatically be related to them. But brain fog can be due to other reasons, so it is worth having a conversation with your doctor about it and any other symptoms to see if further investigations are needed.

What are some lifestyle tweaks we can try to help with it?

As always, lifestyle factors are important: focusing on improving your sleep with techniques such as good sleep hygiene can be helpful (see p.135). As can ensuring that you eat a healthy diet and move your body regularly, as well as stopping smoking, limiting alcohol, and reducing your caffeine intake.

Recognizing your limits and setting boundaries can help to reduce stress, which can be effective. Ensure that you take time to do things you enjoy, and allow time for your mind to rest (see pp.141–143). Psychological therapies can also be useful (see pp.38–41).

What about medical treatment options?

Treatment options will depend on the cause of the brain fog. For example, if it is a side effect of a medication, then the medication may be altered; if it is related to depression, then treating the depression can improve the symptoms.

While HRT has not been shown to be effective in treating brain fog relating to the menopause, if the brain fog is due to insomnia from hot flushes or low mood related to the menopause, then HRT may help to treat these, and therefore the brain fog in turn.

DEMENTIA

When I was experiencing brain fog, my biggest worry
was that I was going through early-onset dementia.
Forgetting words, not remembering where I'd left things,
and finding it hard to concentrate were some of the most
concerning symptoms. I would try to find ways to cope
with these memory blips, such as putting reminders in my
phone or leaving scribbled notes by my bed. After four
anxious years I decided to speak to a specialist, which is
something I wish I had done earlier as it was a huge relief
to hear that I had nothing to worry about. But how do we
recognize the difference between brain fog and dementia?

Q & A
Professor Guy Leschziner, Consultant
Neurologist and Professor of Neurology

What is the difference between the symptoms of brain fog and dementia?

It's very unusual for brain fog to be the
first feature of dementia. The cognitive
processes that occur in the early stages of
dementia are not just difficulty thinking or
clarity of thought, it is usually the loss of
autobiographical memory, getting lost in
places that should be incredibly familiar,
or marked behavioural changes such as
change in personality. It's a somewhat
different clinical picture of brain fog, but
if you are concerned then see your doctor
to check if there are any strong features to
suggest that this is something other than
perimenopause. If so, get a referral to a
neurologist or another cognitive expert.

What are the risk factors for dementia?

Our genetics and lifestyle can impact our
risk. Having a parent with Alzheimer's
disease increases your risk of developing
the disease significantly. However, one
of the biggest risks for exacerbating
conditions like Alzheimer's or other forms
of dementia is the compromise of the
blood vessels supplying oxygen and
nutrients to your brain and removing

waste. This is why conditions like high blood pressure and diabetes, as well as behaviours such as smoking, increase the risk of cognitive decline.

Does oestrogen help to protect us?

The current data is not conclusive. (For more information on the benefits of oestrogen, see p.47.) For now, we have to rely on brain MRI research, short-term clinical trials, and carefully controlled observational data to try to unravel the dementia conundrum.

What should you do if you've been diagnosed with early-onset dementia?

If you have been diagnosed by your doctor, it's important to make sure you are seen by a cognitive specialist to be sure it is actually early-onset dementia rather than anything else. If you are then formally diagnosed with young- (early-) onset dementia, there are a variety of treatments available that will be discussed with you.

What are the treatment options, and is there anything new on the horizon?

It's important to note that not all dementia is Alzheimer's disease, so treatments may be specific to the underlying cause of your dementia. There are a number of drugs that can help improve cognition in the early to moderate stages of the disease, and there are some antibody treatments that have recently been developed which directly target the protein that is thought to be responsible for Alzheimer's disease. These are being used in specific clinical settings, often in the context of trials, and there are many research studies that you can get involved with, too.

Reduce Your Risk

- Take regular exercise (see pp.120–131).
- Control and check your blood pressure.
- Don't smoke as smoking is a big risk for vascular disease of the brain.
- Don't drink too much, try to abide by government guidelines (less than 14 units a week), although some studies suggest that abstinence is ideal.
- Keeping socially active or taking up new skills such as painting, learning an instrument or a new language, writing a book, or doing a crossword puzzle can all help reduce your risk of developing dementia.
- Stay connected, as maintaining social networks is important, as is dealing with any obstacles such as hearing loss.
- Diabetes is a risk for vascular disease so control blood sugar and maintain a healthy weight (see pp.110–114).
- Get a good night's sleep (see pp.132–139): a growing body of evidence links sleep and long-term cognitive decline.

HEADACHES AND MIGRAINES

Lots of women experience headaches or migraines during midlife and menopause, some for the very first time in their lives. This is quite often due to the day-to-day stresses of juggling all the different demands placed on us and/or our changing hormones.

It can often be hard to distinguish between a headache and a migraine, and therefore not always straightforward to treat. The difference for most women lies in the severity of the symptoms. Most headaches range from a dull to an acute pain, with many of us complaining of feeling pain across our foreheads or pressure on either side of the head. The pain can be tiring but we can usually treat it with rest and over-the-counter medication such as paracetamol or ibuprofen.

Migraines, on the other hand, are often debilitating, with severe throbbing pain, and tend to occur on one side of the head only. Millions of women are impacted daily by migraines, but only a tiny per cent are accurately diagnosed or given appropriate care. Hannah, an advertising Account Director, told me:

I started suffering from horrendous cluster headaches out of the blue at the age of 48. One night I actually went to hospital in an ambulance as I thought I was having a brain aneurysm because it was so bad! The hospital referred me to see a neurologist, but the waiting list was so long it took 18 months before my first appointment.

It was one of the most painful and scary things I've ever experienced and would wipe me out during the days to a point where I was unable to work. I was terrified it would happen while driving and I became a nervous wreck.

HANNAH, 51

Q & A
Professor Guy Leschziner, Consultant
Neurologist and Professor of Neurology

Do our hormones cause migraines?

Migraines can most definitely be affected by fluctuating hormones. Women are much more likely across the board to suffer from migraines than men. A sizeable proportion of women with migraines find that they get much worse at a particular point in their menstrual cycle. It's very common for women, particularly during menopause, to see either a significant deterioration in migraines or actually to develop them for the first time. There are, however, some women who say that their migraines improve after the menopause.

Can adjusting our lifestyle help to reduce the risk of migraines?

If your migraines are very intermittent, there are some lifestyle factors that you can undertake to try and improve your migraine control.

- Avoid changes in your environment, such as light and noise, which sufferers don't respond well to.
- Eat regularly, and make sure that you're not dehydrated.
- Try complementary therapies, such as magnesium supplements: some show evidence of improving migraines.

What medications might help?

Try taking a standard painkiller as an abortive therapy: ibuprofen, aspirin, or paracetamol should be taken as soon as you feel the migraine coming on because it's much easier to treat in the early stages than when it's fully established. For frequent migraines, a range of drugs can be enormously helpful in reducing the frequency or severity. Prescribed medications include amitriptyline, candesartan, propranolol, and topiramate. There is also limited evidence to suggest magnesium, riboflavin (vitamin B2), and co-enzyme Q10 may help.

For those who only have very severe migraines in their premenstrual period (when they're still menstruating regularly) we will very occasionally use the oral contraceptive pill for three months at a time so that the impact of their migraines on their quality of life is limited. We can also use preventative migraine treatments during the premenstrual period in order to try and prevent those migraines from coming on within that window.

For some perimenopausal women, HRT can cause a dramatic improvement in their migraines, but in other women HRT can actually worsen them.

Reproductive & Pelvic Health

I hear from so many women who have suffered or are still suffering with a whole variety of reproductive and gynaecological concerns. Even though they have been to their doctors, they are still confused and concerned, looking for answers and wanting to know what is normal, what isn't, and what their treatment options could be.

UNDERSTANDING REPRODUCTIVE HEALTH

When I look back at my own reproductive health journey, it is littered with gynaecological challenges. It was during my mid-20s, when trying for a family, that problems began to crop up. An early unexplained miscarriage was pretty devastating, and when we decided to try again it became increasingly difficult as my periods were irregular, and I eventually discovered that I had polycystic ovaries.

I was treated with Clomid to help regulate my cycle and induce ovulation, making trying to conceive easier. And a nerve-racking year later I was finally full-term and fully dilated, but faced with the worrying frown of my doctor announcing that he was having trouble locating the baby's heartbeat. I was rushed into theatre and thankfully my beautiful baby girl was safely delivered into my arms.

I went on to have another three children without too many difficulties (all via Caesarean birth due to complications from the first birth), and just before my fourth child was born my doctor asked if we intended to have any more. When we said no, he asked if I would like tube ligation, more commonly known as having your "tubes tied". We decided it would be a sensible option for contraceptive purposes.

Although it was the right decision for us, it may not be for everyone, and it's so important to make sure that all of the benefits and risks (both short and long term), for any gynaecological procedure are discussed with your healthcare provider and ideally someone close to you who can offer some moral support.

I didn't expect that having so many Caesarean births, which left me with a lot of scar tissue, would cause me to develop adenomyosis (where the tissue from the lining of the uterus grows into the uterine wall causing heavy periods, cramping, and sometimes painful sex).

Had I known all of this, I would have been far more prepared and had a clearer idea why I went through early menopause at the age of 43, and why at 49 I would need a full hysterectomy due to extremely heavy periods (the Mirena coil wasn't an option for me due to the amount of scar tissue). I was absolutely terrified of not just a fifth abdominal operation, but at the thought of losing such a precious organ. The emotions wrapped up in the loss of your womb and the physical and mental recovery afterwards cannot be understated.

I know how fortunate I am to have been able to have such a large family, when so many others haven't been able to, so I count my blessings every day. But looking back at my fertility journey, what is obvious is the lack of information and support that I was offered. I also realize now that so much of what I've been through during my more recent midlife and menopause years was a direct result of all that came before.

FERTILITY

We all know that the definition of fertility is simply the
ability to conceive a child. What we're not told is that
it's not quite as easy as just falling and staying pregnant.
Many of you reading this will have either started, are
hoping to start soon, or have completed your family; then
there will sadly be others who have tried unsuccessfully
for years to get pregnant, experiencing what is known
as "subfertility", which is the failure to become pregnant
after a full year of trying.

   We hear all the time that menopause signals the end of
our fertility journey, so if we are still hoping to conceive
as we approach midlife, our ticking clock seems louder
by the second. But what is the reality when it comes to
fertility after 40, and what options are available for those
still hoping to start a family?

   While fertility is obviously not exclusively a midlife
concern, many women are looking to have children later
in life, well into their 40s. There may also be younger
women who are reading this book, perhaps because they
want to be more proactive as they plan for their future,
so this next section provides a general overview of the
fertility landscape.

> I am 42 years old and, because of polycystic ovaries, tried unsuccessfully for
> a baby for years. Everyone told me I was too old and to give up. Well, I want
> to let you know that miracles do happen, and after a nervous nine-month wait
> I can finally announce the arrival of my beautiful newborn baby!

BARBARA, 42

Q & A
Dr Gidon Lieberman, Consultant
Gynaecologist and Medical Director of Fertifa

How and where does fertilization occur?

There are three things needed for natural fertility: an egg, sperm, and a fallopian tube. At the beginning of each cycle – when a woman is still menstruating – small bubbles begin to appear in the ovaries. These bubbles are called antral follicles, and most (but not all) will contain an immature egg. The antral follicles have been dormant since they were made when a woman was still in her mother's womb.

The fusing of sperm and egg to form the embryo takes place in the fallopian tube. Sperm can live in there for 96 hours, so that's why it is important to have sex *before* ovulation if you are trying to conceive. The embryo then travels down the tube and will hopefully implant into the endometrium (lining of the womb).

How many eggs does a woman produce each month?

In any month a group of follicles will begin to mature, and only the best egg in that group will eventually ovulate. The remaining eggs will die and the following month a new group of eggs will begin to mature. Over a lifetime most eggs are never ovulated. Younger women will have many eggs in reserve, with higher antral follicle count (AFC) than older women. The AFC of a 35-year-old is between five and eight on each side, while a 42-year-old woman may have two or less.

Is it possible to test egg quality?

Egg quality means the ability of the egg to successfully fertilize, relating to its chromosome count and structure, and will vary between eggs. Blood testing for egg quality is not precise and no single test can predict current or future fertility. We can measure anti-müllerian hormone (AMH), which is secreted by follicles, and a low AMH level means a lower number of eggs. The AMH level will not change during the menstrual cycle, but other hormone testing, for example tests for follicle stimulating hormone (FSH) and estradiol (a form of oestrogen made by the ovaries), is normally performed in days two–five of the cycle.

The first noticeable change observed in egg quality is the decrease in fertility in women in their late 30s. The fall in egg quality associated with menopausal symptoms will normally only be felt years later.

Is sperm quality as important?

Yes! A healthy egg is able to "repair" some aspects of decreased sperm quality (though the converse is not the case), but as egg quality ages, their ability to repair sperm decreases. This means that sperm quality becomes more important with increasing female age.

Is there anything we can do to improve sperm and egg quality?

Although there is much well-meaning advice available suggesting that changes in diet or use of supplements can improve egg quality, there is no strong evidence that this works. Remember that eggs have been in the ovaries for a lifetime and influenced by many environmental and nutritional agents. However, sperm are constantly renewed and are more likely to respond to improvements in lifestyle and nutrition.

How do female reproductive hormones affect fertility and the menstrual cycle?

Oestrogen is the main hormone produced before ovulation (the release of an egg from one of the ovaries, which is generally about two weeks before the start of menstruation). After ovulation both oestrogen and progesterone are released, and this post-ovulatory phase is always 14 days. These two hormones are needed to stimulate endometrial growth and prepare for implantation of the embryo. If an embryo does not implant then these hormone levels fall, the endometrium will not be stimulated, and it will fall away as a menstrual period.

Why do women become less fertile as they age?

Female fertility is dependent on egg number and egg quality. A woman is born with all the eggs that she will ever have. The better-quality eggs are released early in her reproductive life, and as she ages the pool of good-quality eggs falls, resulting in an ever-decreasing number of eggs capable of making a healthy pregnancy. So in a woman's late 30s to early 40s both egg count and quality are significantly decreased. Female fertility is therefore very age dependant. Women under 30 have about 25% chance of getting pregnant naturally each cycle, falling to 20% for women over 30. If you are 40, then the pregnancy rate is 5%.[13]

If we are having regular sex every month at the right time, why are we not getting pregnant?

For conception to take place you need healthy sperm, eggs, and at least one open fallopian tube, and problems with any of these could cause a delay. If you are worried about not being able to conceive for any reason, then you should speak with a medical professional. If there are no background problems (for instance irregular periods) and you are under 35, then it is generally advised to try for a year before seeking help. If you are older than 35 you may want to look into investigations after six months.

What does a full fertility check entail?

In order to fully evaluate both partners to reach a diagnosis, your doctor will include a semen analysis, confirmation of ovulation, fallopian tube testing, and assessment of ovarian reserve. It may be that no issues are identified during this evaluation, however, many couples (40% or more) will have identifiable male and female factors. In approximately 20% of couples there will be no abnormal test results, and this is known as "unexplained subfertility".

What are the different treatment options for fertility?

For those who are struggling to get pregnant, once you have been investigated for all the possible reasons, a focused treatment plan can be made and your doctor will discuss which course of action is best for you.

The only option that can change egg quality is using egg donation. Although not the ideal first choice for many women trying to conceive in their 40s, using egg donation is a very successful treatment – and the success rates are high (50% or

more), compared to the relatively low success rates of IVF using a woman's own eggs in her 40s – at age 42 the chance is less than 10% per cycle.

IVF complications are more frequent in younger women, when the ovaries are more likely to be very sensitive to medication, resulting in Ovarian Hyperstimulation Syndrome (OHSS), which is far less common in older women. Physical complications with IVF are very rare and relate to accidental damage to the bowel or bladder during egg collection, though the emotional and psychological burden is important to be aware of, too, and support from friends, families, and counsellors is vital.

Treatment Options

- Keep trying for pregnancy naturally with support and advice
- Surgery (for endometriosis/fibroids/fallopian tube problems)
- Medication (such as Clomid or letrozole) in order to correct ovulation problems
- Intrauterine insemination (IUI) with partner or donor sperm
- In-vitro fertilization (IVF) or Intracytoplasmic Sperm Injection (ICSI)
- Egg donation
- Surrogacy

What is egg freezing?

It is a method of preserving a woman's fertility, saving one month's supply of eggs so that she can try and have children in the future. It usually takes around two to three weeks to complete, and will normally involve taking drugs to boost egg production and help the eggs mature. When they're ready, they'll be collected under general anaesthetic or sedation.

Instead of mixing the eggs with sperm (as in conventional IVF), a freezing solution will be added to protect the eggs. When you want to use them, the eggs will be thawed and those that have survived intact will be fertilized with your partner's or donor's sperm. In the UK eggs can be stored for up to 55 years.

Who is a good candidate for it?

You might be considering freezing your eggs if you have a medical condition, or need treatment for a condition, such as cancer, that will affect your fertility; or because you are worried about your fertility declining but are not ready to have a child yet.

If you're a female transitioning to a male, you may also want to preserve your fertility before you start hormone therapy or have reconstructive surgery. Whatever your reasons, it's important to consider egg freezing before the age of 35 ideally, because egg quality begins to fall gradually from 35, with a greater rate of decline from 37.

How can pregnant women stay well?

It is important to ensure that your physical and mental health is as good as it can be as pregnancy puts additional demands on the body, especially heart, lungs, liver, and kidneys. Problems such as pre-eclampsia (blood pressure and kidney stress) are more likely with pregnancy in your 40s, but most women who conceive in their 40s have few health issues. You should discuss your future pregnancy plans with your doctor or obstetrician, and don't forget to take folic acid supplements.

How can we manage our fertility expectations?

It can be a difficult and often frightening situation for women struggling to conceive after 40, and many will feel a mix of emotions ranging from anger to sadness and regret. A good physician will understand this and do all they can to fully evaluate both partners and explain clearly what your options and chances of conception are without raising any unrealistic hopes.

If all avenues have been explored, many people will be offered counselling. Acknowledging your emotions about not being able to have children is an important step in working towards acceptance. Some people choose to look into adoption, whereas others learn to live with, plan for, and eventually embrace living child-free.

MENSTRUAL HEALTH

While concerns around fertility over 40 are a common theme of discussion among The Latte Lounge community, questions about menstrual health absolutely flood our social channels and inbox on a daily basis. So what happens to our menstrual cycles as we age?

The average menstrual cycle runs for 28 days, some shorter (23), some longer (35), but when it comes to menstrual health in midlife, we are no longer just focusing on the length of a cycle, but the effect of our changing flow on our physical and mental wellbeing.

So many women suffer with heavy, irregular, or painful periods, or perhaps notice that their periods are getting shorter or heavier during midlife. This can hugely impact our ability to function normally on a day-to-day basis, which was the case with social worker Yvonne.

I'm 46 and have been dealing with painful heavy periods since I was 14. I am going through perimenopause, and I feel pretty alone in a house of sons and a husband. The most annoying thing for me in this part of life is that my periods can now be quite irregular.

I have been to see a menopause specialist and she assures me that I am 'normal' and that it's most likely due to a small fibroid, but the irregular periods catch me out sometimes. Because my periods are extremely heavy, painful, and more frequent, I was told to get a hormonal IUD – with no discussion of anything to do with menopause. I feel quite full of rage about this, and rage and irritability seem part of who I am now.

YVONNE, 46

Q & A
Dr Gidon Lieberman, Consultant
Gynaecologist and Medical Director of Fertifa

What are the stages and symptoms of a normal menstrual cycle?

Menstruation is the womb lining (endometrium) becoming unstable as progesterone and oestrogen levels fall. We count the first day of the cycle as being the day you wake up with a full flow, and most women will menstruate for between two and five days.

The days before ovulation are called the follicular (or pre-ovulatory) phase, followed by the luteal (post-ovulatory) phase. The luteal phase is always 14 days under normal circumstances, so in a woman with a 32-day cycle her follicular phase is 18 days, during which ovulation takes place.

Changes in the body's hormone levels before a period can cause some women to experience a range of emotional and physical symptoms, some with more severity than others: these include feeling bloated, breast tenderness, mood swings, acne, and loss of libido. These symptoms usually improve when your period starts or a few days after.

Menstrual Cycle Stages

1. As an egg matures, the lining of the womb thickens due to increasing levels of oestrogen being produced by the dominant follicle.

2. Once a peak oestrogen level is detected by the pituitary gland (in the brain), luteinizing hormone is released, causing the egg to be ovulated.

3. The follicle starts to release another hormone, progesterone, which maintains the endometrium in preparation for embryo implantation.

4. If conception does not take place then the hormone levels fall, and bleeding begins on day one.

What happens to the menstrual cycle, and to our ovaries, as we age?

The menstrual cycle is controlled by hormones released by the ovaries and brain (specifically the pituitary and hypothalamus). Ovarian functioning decreases with age because of the fall in egg number and quality, and the release of oestrogen and progesterone becomes erratic, leading to bleeding problems. There is unfortunately no way of improving egg quality, but if your periods are problematic because of hormonal irregularities then medication and/or improving your general lifestyle can be used to balance the levels.

Additionally, thyroid dysfunction is more common as we age and can cause heavy or irregular periods. Menstruation is also affected by any changes in the womb, such as fibroids, endometriosis, and polyps, which also become more prevalent with age.

FIBROIDS

These are benign tumours of the womb that grow throughout a woman's life, reaching their maximum size in the late 30s to early 40s. They can then start causing all sorts of menstrual problems, including irregular, heavy, and painful periods. Fibroids can also grow quite large, causing pressure on the bladder and bowels.

If you don't have any symptoms, or you only have minor symptoms that are not affecting your day-to-day life, then treatment may not be necessary as fibroids often shrink after menopause and symptoms will either ease or disappear completely. If symptoms are impacting your quality of life then it's important to discuss treatment options with your doctor.

POLYPS

These are folds of endometrium that are usually benign but can cause problems, and tend to be more common among women in their 30s and 40s. If they do not pass by themselves then minor surgery can remove them.

ENDOMETRIOSIS

This is a condition where the lining of the womb grows outside of the womb cavity. The resulting problems depend on where the endometriosis has spread: adenomyosis is in the muscle of the womb and can cause very severe period pain; endometriomas, or "chocolate cysts" are cysts of endometriosis in the ovaries; peritoneal endometriosis are deposits on the surfaces of the abdominal cavity.

Very rarely we see endometriosis in tissues far away, like in the lungs. Or it can be present in the scars after keyhole surgery or Caesarean birth. There are many causes of endometriosis, and it can run in families. A wide range of treatment options are available, from medication to surgery. Endometriosis is also one of the major causes of subfertility.

I have suffered with endometriosis and fibroids most of my life, and after numerous laparoscopies I opted for an ablation to try and deal with the very heavy bleeding and painful cramps I was experiencing.

When this didn't help, I was sent for tests by my gynaecologist, who said I was suffering with something called adenomyosis. As I had already completed my family, he recommended a hysterectomy – full removal of my womb, including my ovaries.

NIAMH, 57

When should women seek help with menstrual problems?

Changes in the menstrual cycle are normal with age. If your bleeding is affecting your quality of life, or you are experiencing pain that means taking time off work or which doesn't settle with over-the-counter painkillers, then you should definitely speak with your doctor or gynaecologist. Erratic bleeding or bleeding after sex should also be checked out.

What are the treatment options to deal with erratic bleeding?

NUTRITION
The first thing is to maximize diet quality. If you're not vegan or vegetarian, you can eat good-quality proteins from meat and fish; if you are, try to maximize the protein and iron in your diet. If you're taking iron supplements, it's important to take them with vitamin C because that increases the absorption (see pp.110–114).

OTC MEDICATION
There isn't a great deal you can buy over the counter to help with heavy periods. While the non-steroidal anti-inflammatory medications (such as ibuprofen) are good for pain, they are less helpful for heaviness. The progesterone-only pill (mini-pill) is also available without a prescription in the UK.

MEDICAL TREATMENT
Your doctor will likely check for anaemia and thyroid function, which might need medication. A pelvic ultrasound will look for polyps and fibroids. A first-line medication called tranexamic acid is often very helpful in making periods lighter and will not affect fertility.

HORMONAL TREATMENT

This might be using the combined oral contraceptive pill, progesterone-only pill, or a hormonal coil (such as Mirena).

SURGERY

If dietary tweaks and medication aren't good enough, we will look at surgical options. Endometrial polyps can be diagnosed with ultrasound, and surgery to remove them will take around 20 minutes. Some women will be able to have the procedure without anaesthetic while others prefer to be asleep.

Fibroid surgery will depend on the location, number, and size of the fibroids. Surgery can be performed from below, with a narrow telescope passed into the vagina and through the cervix (called hysteroscopic), or through the skin by keyhole surgery or a cut (like a Caesarean birth scar). Fibroids can also be treated by stopping their blood supply, which is known as uterine artery ablation and is done by radiologists.

If there are no fibroids then other minimally invasive techniques can be considered including ablation (burning the lining of the womb). The final option is removal of the womb (hysterectomy).

What advice would you give to women considering surgery?

There is no right answer or one solution for every woman, and all options should be discussed. It is important to take time making your decision, and only go forward once you are happy and feel fully informed.

There are lots of good resources online, but stick to official websites such as the NHS and NICE (the governing regulatory body). Although less invasive procedures tend to have fewer complications, all surgery comes with some degree of risk. Make sure you are aware of the potential complications.

At what age can we stop using contraception?

It's not very often that women over the age of 45 or 46 conceive, and when they do conceive, the real issue is that they are likely to miscarry. This doesn't necessarily mean it will happen to you, but you should be aware of the risks and discuss with your doctor. Ongoing pregnancies after the age of 45 are rare, but the official recommendation is that women under 50 use contraception for two years after the last natural menstrual period, one year for women over 50. If menopause cannot be confirmed, contraception should be continued until age 55.

However, it's important to remember that everybody who's having sex with a new partner needs to use barrier contraception and safe sex techniques because sexually transmitted diseases such as chlamydia, gonorrhoea, syphilis, non-specific urethritis (NSU), and herpes are increasing in older adults.

PELVIC FLOOR DYSFUNCTION

Have you ever leaked a bit of urine when out running, or when coughing or sneezing? Are you in pain when you go to the toilet? Do you feel like something is hanging low, or not quite right? If so, you are far from alone, but so many of us find it difficult to discuss the more taboo symptoms of perimenopause and menopause (which can also be caused by childbirth and the natural ageing process): recurrent UTIs (urinary tract infections), pelvic floor dysfunction, and pelvic organ prolapse.

It can feel so embarrassing, can't it, to mention these concerns to our partners or friends, let alone our doctors? But please don't suffer in silence. It's not something you just have to put up with, and there is so much we can do to prevent this happening.

The vulva, vagina, bladder, and urethra all age, just like the rest of the body, with changes in hormone levels, the consequences of childbirth, and increasing weight all taking their toll. Urinary incontinence (urgency or "nervous bladder") and stress incontinence (leaking with increasing abdominal pressure, such as during exercise or sex, or when coughing) worsen with age, and urinary tract infections will also become more frequent. Prolapse (weakness of the vaginal wall) becomes more common, leading to discomfort/dragging sensations and problems with emptying the bladder or bowels properly.

There is lots that you can do to help, including maintaining a good weight and exercising.

There is lots that you can do to help, including maintaining a good weight and exercising; try pelvic floor excercises, Pilates, bladder training, and physiotherapy, as well as taking medication to calm the bladder, using medical devices, and surgical options. When it comes to looking after your pelvic health, it is critical that any new symptoms of pain, bleeding, or vulval itching you experience are checked out.

Ever since the birth of my three children I have had so many issues with my bladder control. But as I turned 40, things have got progressively worse, especially in the run up to my period. It's really knocking my confidence and I worry about taking the dog for a short walk now, or even laughing, sneezing, or coughing, and I am struggling to function on a day-to-day basis, including at work. It's just so embarrassing and demoralizing.

AMANDA, 41

When we talk about looking after the health of our pelvic floor we are primarily focusing on the health of our urethra, bladder, vagina, and vulva. You may be one of the many thousands of women who have neglected their pelvic floor over the years, not really giving it much thought until problems start to appear. And that's understandable. But if you are also one of the thousands of women who are starting to experience – or have perhaps suffered for years with – things like stress incontinence, an overactive bladder, sexual dysfunction, constipation, repeated UTIs, or issues with a tight pelvic floor, then there is no time like the present to address them. But so many of us don't even know what or where our pelvic floor is, let alone why it's so important to look after and strengthen it as we age.

Q & A
Jane Simpson, Continence Specialist
and Author of *The Pelvic Floor Bible*

What and where is the pelvic floor?

Your pelvic floor is made up of a group
of muscles that stretch from your tailbone
(coccyx) to your pubic bone and between
the bones that you sit on. These muscles
work a bit like a piece of elastic or a
trampoline, moving up and down as
needed, depending on what it is you are
doing. They can relax so you can pass
urine or open your bowels, and contract
to stop you leaking urine when you cough
or sneeze and to stop you passing wind
in an inappropriate place.

What causes pelvic floor dysfunction?

Childbirth and decreasing oestrogen at the
menopause are the most common causes
of pelvic floor dysfunction. We are living
longer, exercising harder, having babies
later, and will spend about a third of our
lives post-menopause.

Other affecting factors are lifestyle
related: things like constipation, straining
on the toilet, heavy lifting, and a chronic
cough can affect the pelvic floor. There
may also be a hereditary element.

What happens when your pelvic floor is not working properly?

- **Stress incontinence:** this is an entirely
  physical issue, not related to emotional
  stress or anxiety, where you leak urine
  – usually when you cough, sneeze,
  laugh, or run. It may be a little or a lot,
  depending on the severity of the stress
  incontinence. Pelvic floor rehabilitation
  (see opposite) is the way forward here.
- **Overactive bladder:** a feeling of
  urgency or frequency of urine that
  sometimes ends in urge incontinence
  – does the sight of your front door
  make you desperate for the toilet?
- **Pelvic organ prolapse:** see pp.70–71
  for more information.
- **Sexual health issues:** when your
  pelvic floor isn't working properly, it
  can impact your sex life. Many women
  find that they wet themselves or have
  vaginal wind during sex, or find sex
  painful due to vaginal dryness. Often
  too shy to tell their doctor, they stop
  having sex or do it rarely, which can
  put strain on relationships. These
  problems can be sorted out with things
  like vaginal oestrogen, pelvic floor
  rehabilitation, talking to your partner,
  and sometimes vaginal dilators.

- **Constipation:** we like to discuss our bowels even less than our bladder, but we know that 50% of people with chronic constipation do not use their pelvic floor correctly. As constipation can be responsible for making all types of pelvic floor dysfunction worse, it's so important to address this.
- **Urinary tract infections:** a UTI can be unpleasant and uncomfortable, with pain on passing urine, a burning feeling, smelly or cloudy urine, and lower back or abdominal pain. UTIs can become worse or start happening at the menopause due to reduced oestrogen in the vagina and urethra.
- **Tightness in the pelvic floor:** this is when your pelvic floor is unable to relax, which can cause constipation, painful sex, urinary urgency, and pelvic pain. It often goes undiagnosed, so if these symptoms ring a bell, please seek help.

What can be done to help?

Try pelvic floor rehabilitation and bladder retraining, the goal being to retrain the bladder by cutting the number of times you pass urine down to between six and eight in a 24-hour period. Keep a bladder diary to see what you are drinking (we should drink about 1.5 litres per day), and make a note of how often you go to the toilet. Drinking too much tea, coffee, alcohol, and fizzy drinks may make things worse. Try to steadily lengthen the time between your visits to the toilet.

Pelvic floor rehabilitation is key for improving and maintaining pelvic floor strength and health and should be a vital part of all our daily routines.

The exercises are also very easy to do. Try to do them two or three times a day, and find something that you can associate with doing them, like cleaning your teeth, turning on your computer, or driving to work, so you don't forget. It needs to become a habit. If you need motivation to keep going, try the NHS Squeezy app (see p.247), which beeps to remind you when to do your exercises and you can customize it to fit in with your daily life.

Pelvic Floor Exercise

1. Sit on the arm of a chair or any hard surface with your feet flat on the floor, and lean slightly forwards so that your vulval area is in contact with a firm surface.
2. With hands on your thighs, try to lift the area around your vagina and anus away from the surface.
3. Draw up all the muscles at the same time, squeeze, lift, and hold for a count of five (aim to build up to ten). Let go gently and count to five, then repeat the movement again five times.
4. Do ten short, sharp contractions in a rhythmic pattern of squeeze, let go, squeeze, let go, squeeze, and let go.

How else can we improve our pelvic health?

Biofeedback is used in lots of different therapies to gain better awareness of muscle movements. For the pelvic floor, it is usually done using a vaginal device and as you contract your muscles you get a visual response (in a clinical setting, often as a graph on the computer screen). There are now lots of things available to buy that give some element of biofeedback and help with pelvic floor strengthening. Tools and gadgets can be very motivating in our busy lives: vaginal weights, intravaginal devices that work with an app on your phone, small electrical stimulation devices, pants that don't involve a vaginal probe but externally stimulate the pelvic floor. The most important thing is to find what works best for you, and always follow the manufacturer's instructions.

Vaginal oestrogen is a local HRT (applied inside the vagina) that is used to treat the vaginal dryness and irritation that can happen as our oestrogen levels fall during perimenopause, menopause, and post-menopause (see pp.22–23). It comes as a tablet, pessary, cream, gel, or ring and can be prescribed by your doctor in the UK. In some countries it can be purchased over the counter too. This can play an excellent part in your pelvic floor health and pelvic floor rehabilitation.

How to Help Yourself

- Try to maintain a good diet and healthy weight.
- Avoid constipation and straining on the toilet: using a raised footstool can help as it puts you in a slightly squatting position, relaxing a muscle around the back of the rectum.
- Practise regular pelvic floor strengthening exercises.
- Try Pilates and yoga: always ask for the correct exercises to help pelvic floor function.
- Avoid heavy lifting.
- Quit smoking (aside from the many other health concerns around smoking, coughing will not help your pelvic floor).

Pelvic floor
rehabilitation should
be a vital part of all
our daily routines.

—

PELVIC ORGAN PROLAPSE

A complication that can occur if your pelvic floor is not working is something called pelvic organ prolapse. This is when the bladder, the uterus, and/or the rectum start to shift out of their proper anatomical position and bulge either into the front or the back wall of the vagina or, in the case of the uterus, descend into the vagina.

Pregnancy and childbirth are known contributors to the development of pelvic organ prolapse, as are chronic coughing and constipation. During perimenopause and menopause, when we have a decline in oestrogen, tissues in the vagina, around the urethra, and around the bladder become thinner and drier. There's less resilience, which can contribute to less support, and this can exacerbate a pre-existing prolapse or cause one to develop.

Q & A
Kim Vopni, Pelvic Health Physiotherapist
and Author of *Your Pelvic Floor*

Can we prevent prolapse?

We absolutely can prevent pelvic organ prolapse. We should be taught preventive strategies throughout our lives. That's not yet happening, but we have the power to start today and pay attention to our pelvic health like we pay attention to the skin on our faces.

The pelvic floor is also the foundation of our core, supporting our spine and pelvis. So we can benefit from pelvic floor physical therapy. I would recommend seeing someone every year, just like we go to the dentist, because early stage pelvic prolapse can be asymptomatic. When it becomes a little bit more advanced, the symptoms can really be quite bothersome.

Symptoms of Prolapse

- Back pain
- Sense of heaviness and dryness in the pelvis, especially as the day goes on
- Feeling like you have something stuck in your vagina
- Difficulty with penetrative sex, with the bulges being uncomfortable
- Difficulty emptying your bladder or bowels
- Struggling to insert a tampon, or tampons can get pushed out

Which treatments and lifestyle changes can help improve prolapse?

The gold standard would be to see a women's health physiotherapist, but if that's not available to you, there are things you can do yourself. In order to test the strength of your pelvic floor muscles, you can insert your own fingers or your partner's into the vagina, or if you have a male parter they could use their penis, and gently squeeze and release to give you an idea of the muscles' strength.

- Avoid constipation and straining on the toilet and work on improving your gut health (see pp.116–119).
- Try Kegels, a voluntary contraction and lift-and-let-go of the pelvic floor muscle. Always ensure you have isolated the correct muscles.

- Use pessaries, which are like an orthotic for your vagina. They are inserted so they apply pressure and support to the walls of the vagina and any organs that are starting to shift out of their position.
- Maintain a healthy weight: being overweight affects all of the muscles in our bodies, but the pelvic floor especially because it's so central and is a bit like a supportive hammock that manages all of the load.

When is surgery the only option?

There isn't really a perfect time to have surgery, and it is not mandatory: people live with stage three and four prolapses, managing them with pessaries, oestrogen, and exercise. But if symptoms are interfering with your life to such a degree that your quality of life has declined, and you have tried all the conservative approaches without success, then this is absolutely a time when you could be considering surgery.

The conservative approaches to helping improve or manage prolapse are important both before and after surgery to ensure that you are in the best possible shape, and you need to do pelvic floor exercises. You must appreciate that there were contributing factors that led to the development of the prolapse in the first place, so you need to make sure that you continue to maintain resilience in those muscles for ever.

Gynae & Breast Cancers

Each year in the UK alone, more than 22,000 women are diagnosed with a gynaecological cancer,[14] which means 60 receive this life-changing news every day. Breast cancer is also a hugely emotive topic, and with media attention focusing on the seemingly alarmingly high rates of breast cancer among women, most of us live in fear of developing it: but to what extent are our fears really justified, and how has the landscape changed in the last 50 years?

GYNAECOLOGICAL CANCER

Often, women might dismiss symptoms such as frequent urination and bloating as nothing to worry about, and in many instances they are right, but sometimes it can be a sign of something more concerning so it's vital to get it checked out. Far too many partners, mothers, daughters, and friends are dying from gynaecological cancers – when quite often some of these deaths could be avoided through better awareness and early diagnosis.

Kathy's story, opposite, is a sobering reminder of why we all need to pay attention to any signs or symptoms that may not "feel right".

I had been experiencing a strange dizziness whenever I sat down. Tests by my doctor didn't show anything worrying, then shortly after I felt a lump in my vagina. I pushed past any embarrassment and asked the doctor for an examination. I was diagnosed with stage 3 vaginal cancer – my tumour was 2.5cm (1in).

During the Covid lockdown, I had a seven-hour surgery to remove the tumour and reconstruct my vagina. The cancer had spread to the lymph nodes, so I had to undergo 25 rounds of radiotherapy and five courses of chemo.

Having gynae cancer can be so isolating, especially when it is so rare and stigmatized. I was at a loss with it all. The average person probably knows about breast and bowel cancers, but vaginal cancer was draining to explain.

Lots of people asked me, 'How did you get that? Did you not go to your cervical screening test?' I'm always happy for people to ask me anything, as it can help to educate people on vaginal cancer. I want women to know their bodies, to talk about their bodies, and to follow their gut reaction if something isn't right. I always say, 'please don't die of embarrassment'.

KATHY, 56

When I set up The Latte Lounge, I was determined to use it as a platform for good in more ways than one and wanted to find a charity partner that we could help to promote and support. The Eve Appeal (see p.248), whose CEO we will hear from next, was a natural fit as the leading UK charity raising awareness of the five gynaecological cancers. The charity saves lives by funding groundbreaking research, which is focused on developing effective methods of risk prediction and earlier detection, and developing screening for all of the gynaecological cancers. Their vision is simple: a future where gynaecological cancer is a disease of the past.

Q & A
Athena Lamnisos, CEO of The Eve Appeal

What symptoms should women be aware of when it comes to gynaecological cancers?

The five gynaecological cancers (ovarian, womb, cervical, vulval, and vaginal) have quite different symptoms, but there are many symptoms that overlap.

OVARIAN CANCER

The ovaries are tiny organs deep within your pelvis. Symptoms of ovarian cancer are quite different to the other gynaecological cancers, and include bloating that doesn't go away and is unusual for you. Women are often talked to about IBS because of the bloating, but it's rare to wake up with something like IBS in your 50s and when you're postmenopausal. It's important to recognize what's normal for you and whether it lasts for three weeks or more than 12 times a month.

Symptoms also include pelvic pain, changes to bowel habits and eating habits, and feeling full much more quickly. Going to the loo more often is something that we hear all the time from people who go on to be diagnosed with ovarian cancer.

Occasionally people have abnormal bleeding, but that is not really one of the symptoms of ovarian cancer.

When should symptoms be checked out?

These kinds of changes, which can easily be confused with other things, are important to get checked out. Go to your doctor, talk about the symptoms, and ask, "Could it be ovarian cancer? Would I be eligible for a CA125?" CA125 is a simple blood test that tests for a raised protein marker; it's not a test to find ovarian cancer but is often used, alongside an ultrasound scan, as an indicator that further tests are required in women who don't have a family history.

What are the treatment options?

The treatment for ovarian cancer has changed considerably over the last five to eight years, particularly with new drugs and PARP inhibitors (a type of targeted cancer drug). We've got much better at surgery, so we're removing the opportunity for cancers to metastasize (spread), like with ovarian cancer, to stop them in their tracks.

WOMB CANCER

This is the fourth most common cancer in women in the UK and the most common of the five gynaecological cancers, with over 9,700 people diagnosed every year.

Its incidence in the UK has increased by 12% in the last ten years.[15] Womb cancer's main red flag symptom is abnormal bleeding (see below). No postmenopausal bleed is normal. Never think, if you're postmenopausal (i.e. it's been a year since your last period), that this is a "last hurrah" period or a final period. That's not normal, and it needs to be checked out.

Can womb cancer be treated?

It is very treatable, so if a doctor refers you under the two-week-wait pathway, you will have a very good outcome. It's not exclusively diagnosed in women postmenopausally, it is also diagnosed in younger women, but it is more prevalent in postmenopausal women.

Gynaecological Cancer Symptoms

OVARIAN CANCER

- Feeling full more quickly or appetite loss
- Bloating that doesn't go away
- Changes in bowel habits
- Needing to wee more often or urgently
- Pelvic pain

WOMB CANCER

- Bleeding after sex, in between periods, or postmenopause
- Blood-stained vaginal discharge

CERVICAL CANCER

- Bleeding after sex, in between periods, or postmenopause
- Pain during or after sex
- Unexplained lower back pain
- Abnormal discharge
- Pelvic pain

VULVA CANCER

- Skin changes in the vulva area
- Persistent itch
- Pain or soreness
- Thickened, raised, red, lighter or darker patches of skin
- An open sore or growth
- A mole that changes shape or colour
- A lump or swelling

VAGINAL CANCER

- Abnormal bleeding
- Blood-stained or smelly discharge
- Pain during penetrative sex
- Internal lump or growth
- An internal itch that won't go away
- Pain when urinating
- Persistent pelvic and internal pain

Do lifestyle factors greatly affect it?

Many womb cancers are oestrogen-based cancers and closely linked to obesity; oestrogen lives in fat cells, and as we get older, fat often collects around our middles. So obesity is something you should address to reduce your risk.

CERVICAL CANCER

We know that 99% of cervical cancers are caused by human papillomavirus (HPV), which we test for in cervical screenings. Most of us are going to come into contact with HPV in our lifetimes through sexual contact, whether that's genital touching or penetrative sex.

HPV is a risk factor for many cancers: vulva cancer, some throat cancers, and anal cancer, not just cervical cancer. Cervical cancer is one of the cancers that we can prevent; you're not even detecting cancer, you're detecting cell changes before they become cancerous.

Is it critical to attend screenings?

We're achieving better awareness of cervical cancer, so people are getting to their doctors more swiftly. However, we do have issues with people not attending cervical screening tests, so cervical cancer remains most common in women under the age of 35 and we need to change that, even though it's not a common cancer in that age group.

There are many reasons why people find cervical screening difficult, but it's so important to attend your appointment.

VULVA CANCER

The unfortunate thing with vulval cancer is people often think, "oh, I've never heard of it, it can't be cancer", even though they know that lumps elsewhere might be cancer. Symptoms include skin changes in the vulva area, patches that, depending on the pigmentation in your skin, will likely to be red, lighter or darker in colour.

You can only look out for skin changes if you know what the skin looks like in the first place, so I encourage people to check their vulva skin monthly. You're primarily looking for lumps and bumps, so it might be you or your partner that spots it. It's important not to self-treat for longer than three weeks without being examined.

Does it mainly affect older women?

Vulva cancer is diagnosed in older women; most of those diagnoses come over the age of 60 and we are seeing growing numbers, possibly because of longevity and for a range of other reasons.

VAGINAL CANCER

This is a very rare disease, and is diagnosed in just over 250 people in the UK each year. It is most commonly diagnosed in people over 60 (with 40%

of cases seen in women over 75) and is rare in people under 40. The incidence of vaginal cancer has remained relatively stable over the last 25 years.[16]

What are the risk factors for vaginal cancer?

The following risks have been identified:
- having had cervical cancer or womb cancer treated with radiotherapy
- a history of smoking
- having a weakened immune system
- human papillomavirus: HPV is present in more than two-thirds of cases, which suggests that it may increase your risk of developing the condition
- abnormal cells in the cervix called cervical intraepithelial neoplasia (CIN), or in the vagina called vaginal intraepithelial neoplasia (VAIN)

VAIN describes cells that are abnormal and are thought of as being in a pre-cancerous condition. It's believed to be closely linked to having a persistent HPV infection, and if left untreated it can turn into cancer.

If you were born with a vagina then you are at risk of vaginal cancer. This is relevant to you if you have not undergone genital surgery; or if you have undergone gender affirmation surgery and some of your vaginal wall was remodelled during a metoidioplasty, or vaginal tissue was left or remodelled during a phalloplasty (both procedures are sometimes referred to as "bottom surgery").

Manage Your Risk of Gynaecological Cancers

- Know your family history
- Recognize the signs and symptoms
- Get to know your body: understand what's normal and what's not for you
- Don't smoke
- Maintain a healthy weight
- Attend regular cervical screenings

What can women do to reduce risk?

Know your family history. You don't inherit cancer, you inherit a risk of cancer development. If you know that you're at high risk because you carry a genetic mutation – which might be BRCA1 or BRCA2, or Lynch syndrome – understanding what that means and what steps you can take to reduce and manage your risk is vital. Reducing your risk could mean having surgery to remove the affected organs, attending regular screenings, making lifestyle changes, or just being aware of changes in your body and getting these checked out early.

It's important to be vigilant and keep track of your hormonal and menstruation history. Understand what's normal for you in terms of bleeding, what is abnormal in terms of your periods, and if you are postmenopausal keep a date of your last

It was shortly after my father had tested positive for the BRCA1 gene that I found out I was also a carrier, at the age of only 23. I was told that at some point it would be advisable to have a double mastectomy, but that I didn't need to rush into anything as I was very young. But they said they would still want to test me annually. At 27 I finally decided to go ahead with the procedure, followed by a reconstruction.

I now have biannual ultrasound tests to check the health of my ovaries too, and I have been advised that if I haven't finished my family by the time I'm 40, I should consider freezing my eggs and have a total hysterectomy to prevent ovarian cancer.

I want people to be aware that, as in my case, the BRCA gene can go through the father's side, and that men can also get breast cancer. But please don't be scared – if you think you may have a genetic risk in your family, go and get tested as soon as you can.

HAYLEY, 31

period. It's also crucial to get to know your body generally: what's inside your pelvis, how you feel; what's normal for you in terms of how often you go to the loo, and when you get full.

What lifestyle changes might help?

There are all of the general hygiene factors – smoking's not great for anything, and it's definitely not great in the way that it interacts with human papillomavirus. With vaginal, cervical, and vulva cancers (HPV-related cancers), smoking is a key factor for helping HPV do its nasty best,

so try to stop smoking. It's vital to maintain a healthy weight, which we know is not easy during menopause when fat cells can accumulate around the middle, but as womb cancer, and to an extent ovarian cancer, are oestrogen-related, it's really important to be aware that being overweight increases risk.

What should I do if I'm worried about being high risk due to family history?

If you're worried about family history, talk to your doctor. Or contact Ask Eve at the Eve Appeal (see p.247) if you feel like you really don't know enough about whether what you have could be defined as a "family history". Finding out that you are at high risk of developing any disease isn't easy to process, especially if it's information that you will need to communicate with your wider family, including your children and siblings, and potentially your cousins and parents too.

Are there any preventative treatments?

This is something that really needs to be talked through with your team to discuss what action to take, because preventative surgery, depending on your life stage, is very, very different for different people.

It might include a double mastectomy, or having your ovaries and fallopian tubes removed. Or it might be a hysterectomy, and if you haven't had your family or completed your family that leads to a number of decisions. A double mastectomy is not an easy decision in itself: the implications are profound. But there are lots of great networks out there that you can speak to.

Although frightening, knowledge is power, and preventing every single case of cancer that we can is important. It's important information for you to have so you can make a personal decision about where you want to go with it. If you come from a high-risk community, for example if you're of Jewish descent, you can be tested now on the NHS with no family history.[17]

What are the considerations around HRT and cancer?

HRT is not for everybody, but it can be extremely helpful for many. I'd encourage everyone to look at the facts and figures, so they really know and understand their own personal risks (and see pp.22–23).

When it comes to cancer diagnosis and whether to take HRT, you need to understand unopposed progesterone and oestrogen (the two hormones work together, so an imbalance in one causes the other to become "unopposed"). If you haven't got a womb, it's crucial to realize how important oestrogen is: if you've had a full hysterectomy, where your ovaries have been removed too, you only need the oestrogen part of HRT. If you do have a womb, you need both oestrogen and progesterone to protect the womb lining.

What are the aims of the Eve Appeal going forward?

When it comes to research funding, cancer research is one of the best-funded health causes in the UK. But gynaecological cancers are a pinprick, with less than 6% of medical research funding going towards prevention and early diagnosis.

We know that prevention is better than cure, and that's why the Eve Appeal's focus on raising awareness and funding is so important, in order to make things better for any girl born today so they should face a different future.

BREAST CANCER

I bet there isn't a single reader here who hasn't at some point known someone who has been diagnosed with breast cancer, or, like me, lost a good friend or family member to the disease. Breast cancer is a topic that is incredibly close to my own heart. My father, the retired British Surgical Oncologist Professor Michael Baum, was awarded the prestigious St Gallen Biennial Prize for lifetime achievements in breast cancer research and treatment to acknowledge his significant contribution to women's health. Together with his colleagues at UCL, Professor Jeffrey Tobias and our next expert, Professor Jayant Vaidya, he most recently pioneered a revolutionary new technique for delivering radiotherapy at the time of surgery for suitable patients, which you will hear more about here.

Q & A
Professor Jayant S. Vaidya, Professor of Surgery and Oncology, specializing in breast cancer

How common is breast cancer, and what are the risk factors?

Worldwide, it's the most common form of cancer among women, with an estimated 2.3 million new cases diagnosed in 2022.[18] In the UK, about 55,000 women are diagnosed annually.[19] Survival rates started improving in the late 1980s.

All modes of treatments have seen improvements, and in the last 35 years deaths from breast cancer have nearly halved.[20] The risk for developing breast cancer appears to be higher when breast tissue, especially the less mature breast tissue, is exposed for a longer period of time to environmental factors that can promote the development or growth of cancerous cells. These include:
- when menstrual periods start at an earlier age and stop at a later age
- when the first pregnancy is later in life
- when breast-feeding is absent or for a shorter duration

With regard to factors that are within our control, the risk is lower in women who take regular exercise, and higher in those who put on weight, especially after menopause. Risk of breast cancer and relapse is higher in smokers, and in those who live in urban areas. Drinking alcohol increases the risk, with no lower limit that is risk free. Eating more fruits, vegetables, and nuts and reducing fat intake reduces the chance of dying after breast cancer.

To what extent is breast cancer genetic?

The risk is higher when a woman carries a mutation in one of the breast cancer susceptibility genes such as BRCA1, BRCA2, and others that normally repair potentially dangerous DNA damages. The chance of mutation is higher in certain populations (those with Jewish particularly Ashkenazi, Polish, and Icelandic ancestry). These genetic factors are thought to be responsible for about 5–10% of diagnosed breast cancers.[21] Patients with these mutations need to discuss the options with their clinical team, such as regular screenings or surgical options such as bilateral prophylactic mastectomy.

Can HRT or the contraceptive pill increase the risk?

As some breast cancers are dependent upon oestrogen to grow, logically, the risk is expected to be higher in women who take oral contraceptive pills or HRT.

Signs & Symptoms

- A lump in the breast
- Dimpling/change in shape (slight dimpling of the skin, especially after raising arms or bending forward can be an early sign of breast cancer)
- Change in the size of one breast
- Eczema-like skin change of the nipple
- Nipple discharge, especially when it is from a single duct or blood-stained
- Lump in the armpit (axilla), but this is uncommon as the only sign of cancer
- Rarely, new breast pain, especially after menopause, that's persistent and localized to one area
- Sometimes just a feeling of something being not quite right, especially in one breast only

However, the relationship is not so clear-cut. Some women may consider the small increase in risk worthwhile for the sake of the improvement in quality of life they provide (see pp.20–23). The decision about taking these medicines should be a joint discussion with a doctor/specialist.

Are there any risks involved in breast screening?

Breast screening began in the 1990s, when research found that it reduces the chance of dying from breast cancer. The results of new analysis of the older randomized

Kinder and effective
treatments can lead
to a good quality of
life that is much
longer than was
possible even
a decade ago.

—

trials, as well as widespread recognition of the overdiagnosis that results from screening, suggest that the balance between benefit and harm from screening may not be quite so sharply defined. Overdiagnosis means diagnosis of a cancer that may have never progressed in the woman's natural lifetime. It is now well established that some cancers may never grow, yet it is not possible to tell the fatal and non-fatal ones apart. Potential harms from screening include overdiagnosis leading to potential overtreatment, additional evaluations, biopsies that can turn out to be benign (in 9 out of 10 women), and the stress and anxiety of waiting for results.

Do the benefits outweigh the risks?

The benefit of screening is much smaller than what one would have hoped for. For every 10,000 women screened in the UK from age 50 for 20 years, about 681 cancers will be found, of which 129 are estimated to represent overdiagnosis and 552 as those that would have progressed. It is estimated that screening would reduce the chance of dying from breast cancer from 2.13% to 1.7%.[22]

However, this is perhaps the most important point: the existence of a breast screening programme brings with it the infrastructure (including radiological, surgical, radiotherapy, medical oncology, psychology, and nursing expertise), as well as quality assurance mechanisms that improve the treatment of all breast cancers and therefore benefits all women. This substantial effect cannot be underestimated and has probably resulted in much of the reduction in mortality we have seen.

Should we be examining ourselves?

Breast self-examination (done in a specific manner) has been tested in a large randomized clinical trial in China and further studies from Russia and the UK. It was found that women instructed to do BSE did find a few additional cancers (as well as additional non-cancerous lumps) and the cancers they found were smaller, but unfortunately the mortality from breast cancer for the group who did regular BSE was no different from those who did not. Since the results of these trials have been known, the focus has shifted to simply being "breast aware", and if any change is noticed, to seek advice.

A recent randomized trial from India suggests clinical breast examination reduces the incidence of higher stage breast cancer, and can reduce the death rate in women over 50. There is also a suggestion it could reduce overall mortality.[23]

How do you make a diagnosis?

Diagnosis is made by a thorough history, careful clinical examination, imaging such as mammography and ultrasound (and sometimes MRI scan), and tissue diagnosis with a needle biopsy. New methods of diagnosis using artificial intelligence and nanotechnology are showing promise, but are still far from replacing humans.

How is breast cancer treated?

The mainstay of treatment is complete surgical removal from the breast and the armpit. If the breast is preserved, radiotherapy is considered necessary. These treatments on their own are able to offer long-term control/personal cure (where no cancer cells are detectable) to a large majority of patients.

Additional treatment (known as adjuvant systemic treatment) is given for any cells that might have spread to the rest of the body before the cancer was removed. The chance of such a spread depends on the type, aggressiveness, and stage of the cancer, and can vary from 10% (most common) to 40% (less common). Once the cancer has come back in other parts of the body it is unfortunately not curable. Therefore, the systemic treatments are given and can reduce the chance of the cancer becoming fatal by 3–20% in absolute terms.

Surgery is now a lot kinder to women. Over 70% of women in the UK can now preserve their breast.[24] If a lumpectomy removes a large proportion of the breast, then the remaining breast can be remodelled to make it look as close to its previous shape as possible.

Non-Surgical Systemic Therapies

- **Endocrine therapy:** only useful when the BC cells express oestrogen ER and/or progesterone PR receptors. They aim to stop oestrogen from stimulating cancer cells (e.g. tamoxifen), or stop the production of oestrogen in fat cells after menopause (preventing ovaries from working or removing them, or stopping the production of oestrogen in fat cells after menopause). These drugs (e.g. anastrozole) are so remarkably well tolerated that they can be called magic bullets.

- **Chemotherapy:** works by killing fast-dividing cancer cells but also kills other normal fast-dividing cells such as hair, and blood cells in bone marrow. Normal cells recover but cancer cells don't. Managing that toxicity is essential.

- **Biologic therapy:** such as trastuzumab (Herceptin) block the c-ERB2 receptor, which is present in some (about 15%) patients' cancers, killing those cells.

- **Bisphosphonates:** (usually given as a six-monthly injection) change the tumour microenvironment and prolong lifespan.

- **Immunotherapy:** is emerging as a treatment for triple negative breast cancer. It has been shown to reduce the chance of cancer coming back, but not yet shown to prolong lifespan.

LUMPECTOMY

When the breast is preserved, the cancer is removed along with a thin margin of normal breast tissue (wide local excision or lumpectomy). When lumpectomy is chosen, it is considered essential to give radiotherapy to the preserved breast because it reduces the chance of the cancer coming back in the preserved breast. Traditionally radiotherapy (called External Beam radiotherapy, EBRT) is given to the whole breast a few weeks after the operation, a course of daily doses for three to six weeks. In the UK, but not elsewhere in the world, some centres offer radiotherapy over just five days, but such compressed treatment does increase the chance of having a hardened breast and its long-term effects are not yet known.

TARGeted Intraoperative radioTherapy (TARGIT-IORT[25]) is given during the operation immediately after lumpectomy, under the same anaesthetic. Early and long-term outcomes of such a focused way of giving radiotherapy are as good as the long post-operative course of radiation to the whole breast (EBRT), but it is kinder, less painful, cosmetically superior, and much more convenient for the patient. TARGIT-IORT is also safer and can prolong life because it avoids the deaths caused by the scattered irradiation of nearby vital organs such as the heart and the lungs that invariably accompanies external beam radiotherapy.

MASTECTOMY

For those who need a mastectomy, they should be given a choice to either have a smaller and quicker operation with no immediate reconstruction, or to have the breast reconstructed during the initial operation. Each of the options has its pros and cons. Although breast reconstruction may be the preferred option to some, it may not be to others.

Unlike most other treatments for breast cancers, breast reconstruction (or major remodelling of the breast after a large lumpectomy) have not been rigorously tested or proven in a robust way to check whether they improve the quality of life, or are not detrimental to cancer outcomes.

What are the survival and recurrence rates?

Both cancer control and survival rates have been rising in the last four decades. In the UK, on average, 75–85% of women with early breast cancer can expect to live for at least 10 years:[26] the NHS provides a tool that demonstrates how good the prognosis is in many patients with small tumours.[27] With modern treatments, survival for many years has become possible, and kinder and effective treatments, carefully balanced against side effects, can lead to a good quality of life that is much longer than was possible even a decade ago.

Heart Health

The most recent data shows that the increase in women dying of heart attacks is staggering, and with one out of two dying from cardiovascular disease it is now the leading cause of death in women. After the age of 40, more women sadly die in each decade from heart disease than breast cancer, and that difference grows as a woman age.[28]

UNDERSTANDING THE FEMALE HEART

Like so many other areas of health, you don't think about heart disease until you've either personally suffered or know someone else who has. Our main education on heart health, outside of school science lessons, has been via images in the media of older overweight men.

I didn't really get to grips with the workings of the heart until I started suffering with heart palpitations in my mid-40s; these are one of the many symptoms of the perimenopause, but I was terrified that I may be suffering with an impending heart attack. I was referred to a cardiologist, who did a variety of tests but could find nothing wrong. But when I started using HRT, the heart palpitations, along with all of my other troubling perimenopause symptoms, disappeared.

One of the most mind-blowing interviews I have done was for a Latte Lounge online event, "The Midlife Festival", with Dr Philip Sarrel, Professor Emeritus of Obstetrics, Gynaecology, and Reproductive Science and Professor of Psychiatry at Yale School of Medicine in the US. He explained that women, prior to menopause, had very low risk of cardiovascular disease, but after menopause the numbers became equal to men.

EXPERT ADVICE
DR PHILIP SARREL, PROFESSOR AT YALE, US

A major contributor to cardiovascular disease in women is low oestrogen levels due to menopause. The low oestrogen effects on cholesterol metabolism lead to an elevation of the "bad" cholesterol (LDL) and a decrease in the "good" cholesterol (HDL). As a result, there is an increase in plaque build-up in the arteries, making them more vulnerable to constriction induced by adrenaline.

Hot flashes, due to low oestrogen levels, are associated with an increase in adrenaline levels. An indicator of the build-up of plaque in arteries is an increase in calcium in the wall. Oestrogen helps prevent spasm in arteries and reduces the amount of calcium seen in the arterial wall. There are many ways in which oestrogen protects arteries and helps maintain their normal function. The way to reduce risk is to understand the importance of good and bad cholesterol. When women go through menopause they should therefore have a measure taken of LDL and HDL, as about 40% will be very vulnerable.

For those that can and want to take it, HRT in women who are vulnerable can be lifesaving. The earlier you start the better, as evidence shows that it can reduce the risk for osteoporosis and heart disease. However, there's a window of opportunity to take HRT, starting before 60, for reducing the risk of developing cardiovascular disease.

It is important to note that young women who have had a hysterectomy, and who are therefore plunged into menopause instantly, should be given oestrogen-only therapy immediately.

Professor Sarrel indicated that for HRT to stand a chance of helping reduce the risk of heart disease, it ideally needs to be started before the age of 60. But can women gain any benefits from starting it over the age of 60?

According to Consultant Gynaecologist Professor Nick Panay (our expert on HRT and the menopause, see pp. 16–23), there may be more risks in initiating HRT in older women because by that stage the blood vessels have become more atherosclerotic (stiffer with more plaques), and therefore don't respond as favourably to the presence of oestrogen that helps to keep them elastic. There's also more risk of blood clots (thrombosis) and stroke in an older age group. If HRT is initiated in an older age group it should be a lower dose, and ideally oestrogen should be delivered through the skin.

While HRT can be very effective in reducing the risk of heart disease in those who are eligible, there are many lifestyle changes we can and should all be making regardless, to help reduce our personal risks.

Our main education on heart health has been via images in the media of older overweight men.

Q & A
Dr Amanda Varnava, Consultant Cardiologist and Head
of the Department of Cardiology, Imperial College London

What happens to the female heart as we age?

As we get older the heart can become stiffer, which is made worse by high blood pressure (hypertension), by far the most important risk factor that affects women in the early postmenopausal years. During these years blood pressure rises more steeply in women compared with men, and this may be related to the hormonal changes during menopause and weight gain that can occur during this time.

About 30–50% of women develop hypertension before the age of 60.[29] Women who have a family history of high blood pressure or who have a history of high blood pressure in pregnancy are at most risk. Blood pressure should be checked at least yearly (more frequently if there are any risk factors).

Do women's hearts age worse than men's?

The stiffness of the heart can be made worse by type 2 diabetes, and this appears to be more pronounced in women than in men. It's not completely clear why: it may be because of underdiagnosis and undertreatment, or because even if a woman's blood pressure and diabetes are as well controlled as in men, women have a worse response. What we can say for certain is that over the age of 80, there is a higher rate of heart failure in women than in men.[30]

We are all at risk of atrial fibrillation (rhythm abnormality) as we age. The risk is greater with accompanying factors such as high blood pressure and diabetes, and again it is slightly greater in women than in men. Another thing that can happen as we age is that the valves of the heart can degenerate and cause aortic stenosis, one of the most common valve problems. Again, women appear to tolerate this less well than men.

What about cholesterol?

In both genders, the cholesterol that circulates normally in our bodies can start to deposit within the heart's artery walls. This process tends to happen slightly later in women than in men, but from midlife onwards women are not immune. This is often underdiagnosed as women display fewer of the classic symptoms of angina (chest pains) and so their condition is more likely to go untreated.

Cardiovascular Risk Factors

COMMON TO ALL SEXES

- High blood pressure
- Type 2 diabetes
- Smoking
- Family history of premature coronary artery disease
- Obesity
- Inactivity

UNIQUE TO WOMEN

- History of polycystic ovarian syndrome, or PCOS; the metabolic problems that come with this increase cardiovascular risk for chronic disease
- History of high blood pressure in pregnancy or the immediate postpartum period, or of pre-eclampsia; both significantly elevate the lifetime risk for cardiovascular disease
- Premature menopause (before age 45)

What can we all do to reduce our cardiovascular risk as we age?

Lifestyle changes can make a significant impact on lowering blood pressure; these should include:
- reducing salt intake
- drinking no more than 14 units of alcohol a week
- exercising: moderately vigorous for at least 90 minutes each week
- maintaining a healthy weight

These changes can be sufficient to at least delay if not avoid medication. If medicines are required, the most common are calcium blockers such as amlodipine or ACE inhibitors such as ramipril. Both are usually very well tolerated, but can occasionally have side effects such as ankle swelling or a cough, respectively.

An automated home blood pressure machine (with a cuff wrapping around the arm) is useful to self-monitor your health. When checking your blood pressure take at least two readings twice a day for a week. The average of these readings should be less than 135/85, or ideally less than 130/80. If your blood pressure is elevated then please discuss it with your doctor.

What we can all do to try and ward off heart problems as we get older is have regular checks of our risk factors, and cardiologists should also take a history of the conditions unique to women.

What are some of the ways in which the heart can malfunction?

BLOOD SUPPLY
Blockages in the arteries of the heart can be caused by a gradual narrowing due to a build-up of cholesterol, leading to angina (chest pains). If the artery becomes completely blocked this will cause a heart attack, leading to irreversible damage to the heart.

The classic warning signs of angina in men include chest pain, sweating, and breathlessness, but for women the symptoms can be much vaguer and could include poor sleep, sudden lethargy, or pains that radiate to the back, down the left arm, or up to the jaw.

MUSCLE

With every heartbeat the heart contracts and then relaxes. In typical heart failure, there is a problem with contraction (systolic dysfunction), and that presents with breathlessness and swelling of the ankles. It is caused by either repeated heart attacks damaging the heart muscle, uncontrolled high blood pressure, or by inherited genetic heart muscle problems.

A form of heart failure called Heart Failure Preserved Ejection Fraction (HEF-PF) seems to be more common in women, perhaps because it is more associated with high blood pressure and scarring and stiffness of the muscle. The heart still squeezes, but it can't relax. This presents similarly to classic heart failure.

ELECTRICITY

Problems can be caused by the heart beating too fast or too slowly. The latter is a risk factor as we age, requiring the insertion of a pacemaker, but women are not at particularly greater risk than men. However, atrial fibrillation – an abnormal rhythm of the heart, where the rhythm is irregular from beat to beat and often faster than normal – is more common in women. Symptoms are often palpitations, suddenly feeling the heart racing, breathlessness, and sometimes dizziness.

Are perimenopausal and post-menopausal women at greater risk of heart disease?

We don't clearly understand why there's an increased incidence of heart disease post-menopause, but it may be that oestrogen offers some protection. When oestrogen levels drop after menopause, women simply catch up with the trajectory of men, who typically display symptoms of heart disease five to ten years earlier.

What we do know is that until the menopause women have a lower incidence of coronary artery disease (cholesterol narrowing of the arteries) than men, but thereafter they catch up.

Why do so many of us assume heart disease is a men-only issue?

Probably because it is commoner with men in the so-called "prime of life", and therefore receives more attention. There has been a gender bias in all of medicine until relatively recently, and we know that the evidence base has often been only reported in men.

Certainly all the drug trials have historically been done in men. Ostensibly, there were safety issues about prescribing medicines in women due to the possibility they may get pregnant. However we have now moved on, and in America it's now mandatory to have equal gender balance in all of the research studies to address this issue.

How can we reduce our risk of heart disease and stroke?

- **Maintaining a healthy weight** is possibly number one. Not only can obesity lead to higher incidence of heart disease, but also the risks of surgery for these conditions is far higher and the severity of the disease is often greater.
- **Regular aerobic exercise** for a minimum of 30 minutes three times a week, up to 50 minutes five times a week is recommended and protective.
- **Quitting smoking** significantly reduces risk. Chemicals in cigarettes make the walls of arteries sticky and cause fatty material to cling to them, clogging arteries and restricting blood flow, increasing heart attack and stroke risk.
- **Family history:** if you have a family history of premature heart disease (below 60), you need to take action. It's obviously not something you can escape completely, but you can try to avoid what's happened to others in the family by being aware and proactive.
- **Have your lipids checked** sooner than the rest of the population if a parent has high cholesterol and relatives had heart attacks in their 30s or 40s, as there may be genetic high cholesterol, known as familial hypercholesterolemia. Getting tested is very important: you could start on a statin or new therapies to prevent heart disease, stroke, and dementia; your children could be checked, and even started on a statin in adolescence.
- **Know your hormonal history:** if you have been diagnosed with polycystic ovary syndrome (PCOS) your gynaecologist should be recommending regular cardiovascular risk assessment. PCOS is sometimes associated with weight issues, so be mindful of exercise, watching your weight, and checking your blood pressure and cholesterol. Similarly for patients that have had premature menopause, particularly if they didn't go on HRT.

What medical interventions are there?

One is to immediately start on a high dose of statin and tailor your cholesterol results such that your bad cholesterol LDL is to a certain target. That will hugely reduce the risk of stroke and heart attack. For some women at especially high risk, adding aspirin will markedly reduce the chance of a clot blocking the artery and causing a heart attack.

Should we test our cholesterol levels?

I think everyone should have had a lipid/cholesterol and lipoprotein (a) check by the age of 40. But if you've got any of those other risk factors, maybe even before that, and then the frequency of checking your lipids will depend on what that value was and what your other risk factors are.

When oestrogen levels drop after menopause, women simply catch up with the trajectory of men, who typically display symptoms of heart disease five to ten years earlier.

—

Musculoskeletal Health

If there's any symptom that can make you feel old before your time it's the dreaded joint pain. The Latte Lounge is full of discussions about stiffness, aches, and joint pains, whether that's a creaky back in the morning, sore knees, aching hips, painful elbows, or conditions such as arthritis and fibromyalgia. We so often don't understand why we experience "wear and tear" as we age, or what our hormones have to do with it.

JOINTS, MUSCLES, AND BONES IN MIDLIFE

Have you ever made a massive gesture to mark the approach of a big birthday? Perhaps announce to the world that you are going to take up running at the age of 40, or set yourself the challenge of 50 things to do before you are 50? If you are about to set yourself a life-changing target, please don't do what I did and throw yourself into it without preparation or expert advice first.

As I approached my 40th birthday, I decided to take up running, thinking it would be a cheap and healthy way to exercise. All was going well until I felt a shooting pain down the side of my leg, radiating up my back and through my hips, and walking became impossible.

The doctor told me I had slipped a disc (where the soft cushion of tissue between the bones in the spine pushes out of place), and asked if I was aware that I also had hip dysplasia, a condition that, unbeknown to me, I had been born with. Hip dysplasia is seen most often in women, and occurs when the socket in the pelvis, into which the ball-shaped bone at the top of the thigh bone (the femoral head) fits, is too shallow to support it.

Apparently my problems were caused by a combination of constant pounding on the pavements causing a lot of wear and tear (osteoarthritis) in my hip joint, and the hip dysplasia. I was referred to a rheumatologist straight away and temporarily put out of my misery with a steroid injection and referred for sports rehab physio. I was advised to revert to low-impact exercise and to focus on building up my core strength and all-over muscle tone to protect both my back and my hips from future issues.

A couple of years later I started to experience joint pain – another perimenopausal symptom. I would soon understand the impact of low oestrogen on our bones and how weight-bearing exercises and a healthy and varied diet are essential for protecting them from osteoporosis.

I have been in constant pain for the last five years, combined with suffering from extreme fatigue, muscle stiffness, insomnia, headaches, memory problems, and IBS. This isn't just normal pain – even things like trying to put a clip in my hair can make my neck and back go into spasm. No amount of pain relief has helped and after constantly being fobbed off by doctors telling me it was either all in my head or it was due to my lifestyle, at least now I have a diagnosis (of fibromyalgia and perimenopause). But it has and continues to be so debilitating, and it's so frustrating that most doctors don't have a clue how to help me.

WENDY, 49

Although it is not always possible to find total relief from pain, you may be able to reduce it or learn to respond to it in a different way.

—

Q & A
Professor Hasan Tahir, Consultant Rheumatologist,
with Medical Student Mr Syed Haider Tahir

What happens to our joints and muscles as we get older?

Several changes occur in our muscles and joints as we age that can impact our overall mobility, strength, and flexibility. These can include the following.

OSTEOPOROSIS
Most of us will lose bone mass and/or bone density over time, especially women who are going through the menopause. This makes the bone more fragile and susceptible to fractures.

OSTEOARTHRITIS
The cartilage, which is the protective tissue covering the ends of the bones in joints, may thin and become less resilient over time. This can lead to conditions like osteoarthritis, where joints affected include the hips, knees, spine, and thumb.

MUSCLE LOSS
One of the most noticeable changes is the gradual loss of muscle mass known as sarcopenia. With reduced muscle mass, strength and functional capacity may decline. We may also become less flexible and more rigid. These muscle changes usually occur in women at around the age of 40–50.

SHRINKING
As we age, we also appear to shrink a bit. Our foot arch becomes less pronounced, which to a degree reduces our height, and the little gel-like cushions (discs) situated in between each of our vertebrae (located along our spinal column), can become dehydrated, making us seem shorter.

How can we ward against these issues?

It is important to adopt a healthy lifestyle and engage with regular physical activity, including a mix of aerobic exercise, strength training, and flexibility exercises. All of these can help maintain muscle mass, joint flexibility, and overall mobility.

A balanced diet can also support muscle health, and avoiding smoking and excessive alcohol consumption, managing stress, and getting enough sleep are also important factors for maintaining joint and muscle health as you age (see pp.106–167).

Why are women in midlife susceptible to musculoskeletal pain and injury?

Midlife women can experience pain and injury due to a combination of factors, including those related to age outlined above, but also related to hormones. The decline in oestrogen levels at menopause can lead to conditions such as osteoporosis and muscle weakening, as this hormone plays an important role in maintaining bone density and muscle mass.

What common disorders can occur?

Various inflammatory, non-inflammatory, and autoimmune disorders can occur due to the complex interplay of hormonal changes, genetic predisposition, and environmental factors (see box, right).

Is fibromyalgia the most common among women?

This is a long-term condition characterized by widespread musculoskeletal pain, fatigue, sleep, memory, and mood issues. Symptoms often begin after an event such as physical trauma, surgery, infections, or significant psychological stress, but can gradually accumulate over time.

Women are more likely to develop fibromyalgia than men. It is still unclear why some women suffer with it, but it is thought that it is caused by the nervous system in the brain and spine not being able to control or process pain signals from other parts of the body.

How can women distinguish symptoms of the menopause from fibromyalgia?

It can be difficult to discriminate between fibromyalgia and the menopause. These are two distinct conditions, but they can

---

Musculoskeletal Disorders

INFLAMMATORY

- Rheumatoid arthritis
- Psoriatic arthritis
- Axial spondyloarthritis

AUTOIMMUNE

- SLE (Lupus)
- Sjögren's syndrome
- Myositis

NON-INFLAMMATORY

- Fibromyalgia
- Osteoarthritis

---

share some similar symptoms, so it is important to differentiate between them for accurate diagnosis and treatment. Patients with fibromyalgia tend to have tender points and can have symptoms at a young age.

Unlike with fibromyalgia, menopause responds well to HRT. If you are experiencing symptoms that you suspect might be related to either menopause or fibromyalgia, it is important to consult a healthcare professional for a proper evaluation. In some cases, it is possible to experience both menopause and fibromyalgia concurrently, so a thorough assessment is key.

What can help with pain?

Everyone perceives pain in a very different way and so the key is setting expectations to help women understand what we are trying to achieve with pain management.

Education of the underlying condition is fundamental and short-term pain relief such as paracetamol, codeine, and anti-inflammatories can help but are not the long-term solution (see box, right, for pain management options).

Although it is not always possible to find total relief from pain, you may be able to reduce it or learn to respond to it in a different way. Many with chronic pain enjoy a better quality of life if they engage with a pain management programme.

When is surgery required?

Surgery generally has little to offer most with chronic pain. However, patients with conditions such as osteoarthritis, and who have seen no improvement from a pain management programme, may consider seeking a surgical opinion about the possibility of a joint replacement to see if that will benefit them.

Who should we go to see for help?

Start with your doctor, who will then refer you if needed to either a specialist physician or to a surgeon: this might be a rheumatologist – a doctor who deals with musculoskeletal, autoimmune, and

Pain Management

- **Exercise:** a little and often is important for pain management, including stretching, strengthening, and aerobic exercise. Good options include walking, swimming, cycling, and activities such as dancing and Pilates.
- **Physical therapy:** it is helpful to have a supervised regime. This can be delivered by physiotherapists, chiropractors, and osteopaths.
- **Keep working:** it is important to try to stay at work, as research has shown people become less active and more depressed when they don't work, which contributes to their pain.
- **Psychological support:** chronic pain management often needs support from a professional who can help with therapies such as mindfulness and cognitive behavioural therapies (CBT). (See pp.38–41.)
- **Medication:** drugs prescribed for depression and to prevent epileptic seizures have been found to help relieve chronic pain, and offer the extra benefit of treating mood symptoms. These include amitriptyline, duloxetine, and pregabalin. Injections including steroids can also help some patients as part of a treatment plan.

inflammatory conditions affecting any part of the body – or an orthopaedic doctor, who tends to get involved with the surgical aspect of treatment.

Preventative Health Checks

We are all familiar with the old adage that prevention is better than cure, and there are many reasons why it is sensible to keep our health in check after reaching 40, in order to avoid any future problems as we age.

THE ROLE OF SCREENING

There are various screenings and tests available to all that can detect underlying health conditions early on, allowing us to make informed decisions about our lifestyle choices and seek appropriate treatment if needed as soon as possible.

However, it's important not to fixate too much on testing for everything and anything when it comes to our health and wellbeing, especially if you lead a healthy lifestyle and have a good family history; overinvestigation can often lead to unnecessary health anxiety. For more detailed information on women's health screening and tests, please see the relevant chapters in this book and/or speak to your own doctor.

Q & A
Dr Lucy Wilkinson, Doctor and Clinical Advisor
at the online menopause clinic Stella

What is health screening?

Screening is where we check a particular group for a health condition. The idea is to spot potential problems before you start showing any symptoms, allowing for early treatment. This is one of the most effective things that modern medicine has achieved: for example, cervical screening (the smear test) has been saving at least 1,800 lives every year since it was introduced to the UK in the 1980s.[31]

These regular checks are a good way to receive an early warning about certain conditions, but they don't pick up on everything. If you have spotted new symptoms or something just doesn't feel right, you should still see your doctor even if you have had a normal screening test.

If you do not identify as female but were assigned female at birth (AFAB) you still need to attend these check-ups. If you're not automatically called but think you should have been, let your doctor know.

CERVICAL SCREENING

This is a life-saving way to detect early changes that could turn into cancer if left untreated. Cervical cancer is the most common cancer in women under 35 and has a good prognosis if caught early.

Screening currently focuses on identifying human papillomavirus (HPV) infections, which are extremely common. In fact, the vast majority of people who have been sexually active will have encountered this virus, which can be passed on by oral, vaginal, or anal sex. While most people will clear the infection with no further consequences, it will cause changes to the cells of the cervix in a small proportion, and it's these changes that can lead to cervical cancer. Luckily, in most cases affected cells can be treated relatively easily and completely removed.

Currently, all women in the UK are invited for cervical screening from the age of 25 onwards. You should have this done every three years up until the age of 49, and then every five years from 50 onwards.

NHS Screening in the UK

- **Cervical screening:** 25–49, every 3 years; 50–64, every 5 years
- **Breast screening:** 50–70, every 3 years
- **Bowel cancer screening:** 50–74, every 2 years (depends on region, see p.104)
- **NHS health check:** 40–74, every 5 years

Once you hit 65, the NHS recommends that screening only needs to continue if one of your last three smears was abnormal.

Will I need cervical screening during or after menopause?

You still need to have cervical screening if you are going (or have gone) through menopause. This is because, regardless of everything going on with your hormones at this time, changes to your cervix can still happen. Likewise, you need to continue having smears even if you aren't currently having sex.

The only exception to this is if you have had a hysterectomy including removal of the cervix. If this is the case, you no longer need cervical screening.

Are smears painful after menopause?

Menopausal changes to the vagina can make having a smear test tricky. The tightness, pain, and fragile tissues that can be experienced as part of genitourinary syndrome of menopause (GSM, see p.17) can make speculum exams painful or even impossible. If this is the case for you, speak to your doctor for advice.

Likewise, if you're affected by symptoms of GSM in your day-to-day life, they may recommend trying vaginal oestrogen, which is a low-risk and effective treatment available as creams, gels, pessaries, and rings. These can sometimes be used short term in the weeks before your test is due, but should be avoided the night before the test in case it affects your result. Your doctor will advise on whether this is a suitable option for you.

When should I see a doctor?

As well as attending your regular smear tests, you should see a doctor if you have any new or unusual symptoms. This is because screening doesn't test for all of the causes of abnormal bleeding, and you could need further medical tests to ensure that all is well. In particular, seek an urgent appointment if you have:
- vaginal bleeding between periods
- bleeding after sex
- postmenopausal vaginal bleeding
- abdominal pain
- bloating
- changes to your bowel habits
- bleeding from your back passage
- blood in your urine
- needing to pee more often or more urgently than usual
- any other symptoms that are new or troubling you

Smear tests are excellent for screening, but they're often not particularly useful if you have symptoms like abnormal bleeding or pain. If this is the case, your doctor is likely to refer you for other tests such as colposcopy or a pelvic ultrasound.

Cervical screening (the smear test) has been saving at least 1,800 lives every year since it was introduced to the UK in the 1980s.

—

BREAST SCREENING

You will be invited for your first mammogram (a kind of X-ray that can pick up on early signs of breast cancer, sometimes when the cancer is too small to feel), by the time you reach 53 (the NHS sends out invitations between the ages of 50 and 53). You will then be recalled every three years until you reach 71. After this point you will not be recalled automatically, but can request to be booked in for screening every three years.

   If you have a family history of breast cancer or another risk factor, screening might begin earlier for you. If you think this could be the case, ask your doctor.

When should I see a doctor?

You should always see a doctor if you notice any changes to your breasts. These include:
   • breast lumps
   • changes to the size or shape of your breasts
   • skin changes, including dimpling or eczema on or around the breast
   • bleeding or discharge from the nipple
   • lumps in your armpit
   • pain or discomfort

BOWEL CANCER SCREENING

Bowel cancer becomes more common as we age, so it's important to attend screenings when called. Screening has been shown to reduce your risk of dying from bowel cancer.

Breast Screening/ Examination Risks

It is vitally important that you have access to enough evidenced-based information about the benefits and harms of breast screening to make an informed decision. See pp.81–83, refer to the current NHS guidelines (see p.248), and read the Cochrane Report[32] for the most recent research into self-examination. If you still have questions about your own personal risk, discuss them with your doctor.

The age that you'll be invited for NHS bowel cancer screening varies depending on whereabouts you live:
   • 60 in England (50 by 2025)
   • 50 in Scotland
   • 51 in Wales
   • 60 in Northern Ireland

You will be given a home test kit, known as the faecal immunochemical test (FIT), to use. You collect a small amount of poo, which is then sent off to the lab where it is checked for blood. Even very tiny amounts of blood can be detected. As bleeding can be a sign of cancer and precancerous growths called polyps, anyone with a positive test will be invited for further investigations. Bowel cancer can be treated more effectively if it's caught early, and polyps can often be removed as a day case procedure.

Follow-up screening tests then happen every two years. You might be invited for screening earlier or in a different way (by colonoscopy) if you are at higher risk of bowel cancer – for example, due to your family or personal medical history.

When should I see a doctor?

You should see your doctor urgently if you notice:
- changes in your bowel habit (e.g. looser poo or going to the loo more)
- abdominal pain
- bleeding from your back passage
- abdominal swelling or bloating
- weight loss
- any other new or worrying symptoms

This is true even if you have had a recent negative screening test. While screening is helpful, it does not cover all bases. There are many other possible causes for these symptoms that require different tests, sometimes urgently.

THE NHS HEALTH CHECK

This is a general check-up offered by the NHS for everyone aged over 40 to give you an overview of your health, including:
- cholesterol
- blood pressure
- heart and cardiovascular health
- kidney function
- blood sugar levels
- weight and body mass index (BMI)

You'll also be given advice on how to stay healthy in the long term and tackle any risk factors that are present; this could include advice on weight, blood pressure, and diabetes. Any issues identified will be flagged to your doctor, who can then advise you accordingly.

This is particularly important as you go through menopause because some conditions related to these risk factors become more common after this time. You will automatically be called for an NHS Health Check every five years. If you think yours might be overdue, you should be able to book it in yourself by contacting your doctor's surgery.

TESTS DEPENDENT ON HISTORY

Depending on your own medical history, your doctor may advise other screening tests. Examples of these include:
- regular eye and foot checks if you have diabetes
- routine screening tests in pregnancy
- early cholesterol tests if you have a strong family history of heart disease, or familial hypercholesterolaemia

It's also advisable to visit a dentist twice a year to check your teeth and gums.

Screening can be a valuable part of your healthcare, but if you have any new or unexplained symptoms, it's important to get them checked out properly by your doctor as screening tests only look for a handful of specific illnesses.

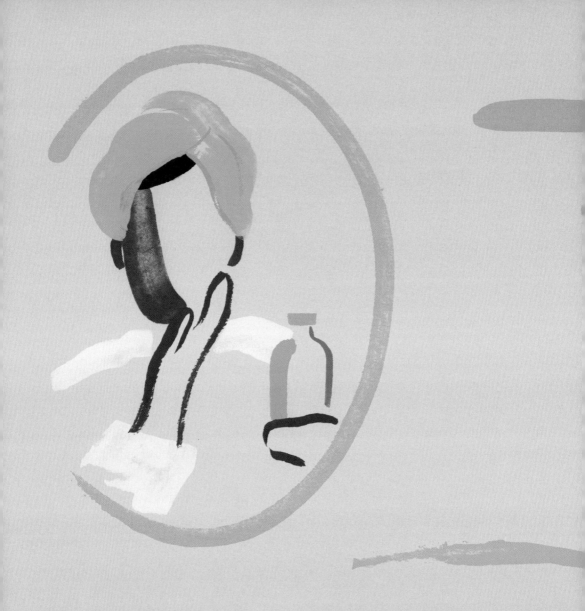

WELLBEING

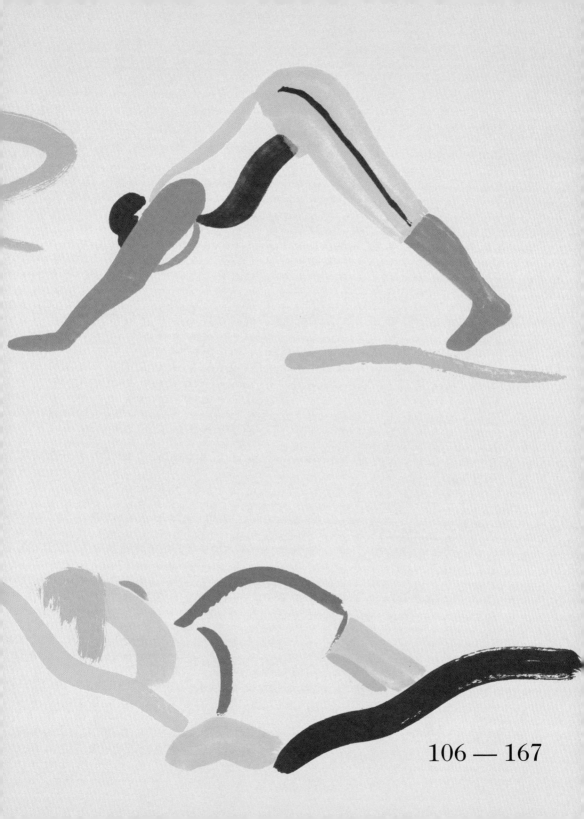

106 — 167

Diet & Nutrition

This is a topic around which there are so many mixed messages, with myriad "experts" advising on foods we should or shouldn't eat. It's no wonder that so many women have reached midlife totally confused about what and how to eat. This section looks at how we can all optimize our diet and nutrition, not just to assist with weight management – one of the most common complaints of midlife – but also to help alleviate some of the mental and physical symptoms of the menopause and look after our long-term health.

HEALTHY EATING IN MIDLIFE

We all know by now that the fundamental purpose of good nutrition is to ensure that our bodies get all the essential nutrients they need to be firing from all cylinders, not just now, but in the long term. But in the confusion of available information, how can we figure out what healthy eating means for us as individuals?

We all have different needs and goals, sensitivities and preferences, and there is never going to be a one-size-fits-all solution, but there are simple tweaks we can all make to ensure that we are meeting our body's changing nutritional requirements.

I am feeling healthier now than I have ever been, since I have incorporated a healthy eating programme designed specifically for menopausal women. The way I eat now has nothing to do with starving myself to fit into a dress and everything to do with nourishing my body for its ever-changing needs and to support my long-term health. My skin is so much brighter, and my energy levels are so much better.

AMBER, 53

I have experienced first-hand how different foods can affect menopause symptoms and sleep quality, and I know how difficult it can be, even if your diet is "on point", to shift those stubborn pounds clinging on to an ever-expanding waistline. Indeed, one of the most commonly asked questions from members of The Latte Lounge community is about how to lose weight during midlife.

One thing I do know is that we are all different. Some of us have really fast metabolisms and never put on a pound, and others, like me, only have to look at cake to put on half a stone. And what worked (or perhaps didn't work) in our 20s and 30s when it comes to weight management is very different to what works in our 40s, 50s, and beyond. It's time to take back some control over our diet, reset, and learn to eat sensibly.

Q & A
Jackie Lynch, Nutritionist, Author, and Founder
of the WellWellWell Menopause Nutrition Clinic

Why is good nutrition so important in midlife?

Our bodies are much more sensitive during the hormonal transition of the menopause, which is why it's more important than ever to get the correct balance of macronutrients: proteins, fats, and complex carbohydrates (fibre). We really should be eating a combination of all three macronutrients with every meal and snack.

Getting these basics right is the single most effective thing that you can do to optimize your health and wellbeing during this tricky phase of life. It's about making long-term changes rather than looking for quick fixes, and thinking in terms of nutritional value rather than calories, which aren't necessarily the enemy.

How is protein essential, beyond building muscle?

Women generally don't eat enough protein. We need protein for strength and stamina, as well as to support bone density and muscle tone. Our bodies are made almost entirely of protein and will prioritize supporting internal organs over hair, skin, and nails, which will suffer if you don't get enough. And the amino acids found in protein-rich foods are required for key neurotransmitters that regulate mood, memory, focus, and concentration.

How can we ensure that we're getting enough protein?

Good-quality protein should form a part of every meal or snack. Some excellent sources include lean meats, oily and white fish, eggs, Greek yogurt, pulses, soya, nuts, and seeds. Don't neglect protein at breakfast: an egg is a great way to start the day, but perhaps not practical if you're in a rush, so consider adding mixed seeds to cereal or porridge, or have protein-rich peanut or almond butter on your toast.

Try to make sure that your lunchtime salad or soup includes lean meat, fish, lentils, or beans, and snack on raw almonds or add hummus to an oatcake. Foods that contain protein also contain fats, so you get double the benefit. Take a look at the box opposite for some ideas on how to boost protein in your meals throughout the day. Aim for a fist-sized portion of a protein-rich food with your lunch and dinner.

Meal Planning

BREAKFAST

- Balance complex carbs, protein, and fats, such as eggs with wholemeal toast or with spinach and avocado.
- Cereal should be wholegrain, avoiding anything with more than around 8g of added sugar per serving.
- Add two tablespoons of pumpkin, sunflower, or ground flaxseed to boost the protein content and add fibre to your morning cereal or porridge.
- Practise portion control: 30g of cereal is ample, so weigh that out a few times and remember what it looks like for future reference.

LUNCH & DINNER

- Make ¼ of your meal protein: healthy options include a salmon steak, a chicken breast, tofu, or a couple of dollops of hummus.
- Complex starchy carbs, e.g. wholegrain rice, pasta, or bread should only make up ¼ of the meal (a fist-sized portion).
- Avoid starchy food in the evening: make ¾ of your meal vegetables instead.

SNACKS

- Eating balanced meals should help you avoid craving snacks, but if needed opt for a protein–fibre combo like chopped veg with 30g of hummus, or fruit with an edible skin and 7 or 8 almonds.

Can fats really form part of a healthy diet?

Fats, together with protein, stabilize blood sugar levels and promote the satiety response, which tells us when we're full. This is crucial if you're struggling with weight management. We're conditioned to believe that fat is bad, but it's vital for our health. Good-quality saturated fat, e.g. grass-fed beef, is used to make sex hormones. Mono- and polyunsaturated fats, e.g. oily fish, flaxseed, walnuts, or avocado, can also help to support cardiovascular health, hormone balance, and optimal functioning of the brain and nervous system.

We're often told to cut carbohydrates in order to manage our weight, but should we be doing this?

Complex carbohydrates are essential macronutrients, rich in fibre, which help to optimize digestion. They also provide a sustained source of energy, which keeps us going for longer, so we're actually less likely to be tempted by snacks. The single best source of complex carbohydrate is vegetables, so try to eat five varieties each day (any fruit can be a bonus on top of that), and ensure that dark green leafy vegetables like kale, spinach, watercress, or spring greens feature every day: these are a one-stop shop of menopause-friendly micronutrients such as calcium, magnesium, vitamin C, and iron.

> *I've put on a huge amount of weight over the last few years and have tried every diet going, but I seem to have a complete mental block when it comes to watching what I put in my mouth. It's like the part of my brain that says, 'you don't need that' switches off, and as soon as I have finished eating it switches on again to ask why on earth I ate it! I feel like I need a boost to get me started losing weight and am considering trying a liquid diet, where I replace breakfast and lunch and then have a meal in the evening. But I know this is not a sensible or sustainable way to eat or to lose weight permanently.*
>
> LIZZIE, 45

Why do so many women struggle with managing their weight in midlife?

Our metabolism slows down at roughly the same time as the perimenopause and menopause. This is related to ageing rather than hormonal changes, and happens to men too, but the timing has a big impact on women, not just in terms of weight gain but also in how it affects body confidence. As hormone levels decline, many women experience low energy and low self-esteem, which makes it even harder to motivate them to exercise, creating a vicious cycle.

What is mindful eating, and can it help with weight management?

Mindful eating is about savouring your food, which is very important. If you rush to eat then your brain won't imprint the memory and you will feel hungry sooner. Taking time over meals, and eating at the table rather than in front of the TV, is an easy way to regulate your appetite. Chewing your food properly means that your digestive system has less work to do in breaking it down, so you won't suffer indigestion and you'll also find you don't eat quite so much.

Should we be cutting sugar out of our diets?

Sugar does play a big part in weight management, and it's important to also be aware that menopause increases our risk of certain conditions, including type 2 diabetes. If you experience blood sugar spikes from eating excessive sugar, your body produces insulin to clear it to the liver to be stored. If you've been eating too much sugar in things like cakes and sweets, this excess will be stored as fat cells, and this can be a fast route to weight gain. Over time you may also risk becoming insulin resistant and eventually diabetic. If you experience dizziness or light-headedness when you stand up suddenly, then eat more complex carbohydrates and protein to help to regulate your blood sugar.

Are "superfoods" worth the hype?

This is basically a marketing term, usually used to describe foods that contain a multitude of nutrients including key vitamins, minerals, and antioxidants. Unfortunately, this can give some retailers the excuse to hike up the price, so it's important to recognize that lots of everyday foods count as "superfoods", even if they're not as fashionable as things like quinoa or maca powder. If you focus on including a range of vegetables in your diet, you'll be getting plenty of crucial macro- and micronutrients.

Superfoods

- Broccoli, kale, and other cruciferous vegetables
- Dark green leafy vegetables
- Berries such as blueberries, cranberries, strawberries, and blackberries
- Sardines and salmon
- Nuts such as almonds and walnuts
- Eggs: high in both protein and nutrients
- Pulses such as chickpeas, lentils, and beans
- Wholegrains
- Seeds, especially chia and hemp
- Flaxseed: a menopause "superfood", containing protein, fibre, omega-3, and phytoestrogens

It's common to feel low in menopause. Can we boost our mood with food?

What we eat and drink can have a profound impact on our mood and mental health. If symptoms persist or are seriously affecting your daily routine, then consult your doctor to rule out a medical condition or see if HRT is suitable for you (see pp.20–23). But there are lots of ways that the right nutrition can help to calm your nerves, boost your mood, and put the spring back in your step. See over the page for some simple dietary tweaks to help with a variety of mood concerns.

Good Mood Diet

- **Maintain blood sugar balance:** low blood sugar can cause anxiety, irritability, and low mood. The best way to balance blood sugar is with a combination of protein and complex carbs with every meal and snack. Our brain is entirely reliant on glucose as a source of energy, and it operates best with the steady drip feed of fuel that blood sugar balance provides.

- **Increase intake of magnesium:** found in leafy green vegetables, almonds, cashews, pumpkin seeds, pulses, and wholegrains, magnesium is nature's calmer. It helps support the nervous system and regulates the body's response to stress. Try juicing spinach, kale, or watercress with apple to sweeten, or try a magnesium double-whammy of cashew butter on a brown rice cracker.

- **Top up on B vitamins:** low levels can contribute to low mood and anxiety, and stress, alcohol, and the oral contraceptive pill can all deplete B vitamins. Vegetables and wholegrains are a good source of B vitamins; egg yolk, meat, and fish are excellent sources of vitamin B3; B12 is only found naturally in animal products, so vegans may need to take a supplement.

- **Limit alcohol and caffeine:** these can affect the delicate chemical balance in the brain, which may lead to low mood over a period of time. Audit your intake to see whether you've become more susceptible during menopause.

Can food boost our energy levels?

Lack of energy is a frequent problem during the menopause. Low levels of iron, vitamin B12, folate, and vitamin D are common causes of fatigue. Foods that contain protein are rich in iron, especially lean red meat, tofu, fish, eggs, and lentils. Complex carbohydrates in wholegrains and vegetables provide a sustained energy source for the body, so a very low-carb diet is not your friend if you're feeling tired. Two handfuls of dark green leafy vegetables every day will support optimum magnesium, essential for the chain reaction of energy production in the body. And remember to drink water throughout the day: just 2% dehydration can reduce energy levels by up to 15%.

Are nutritional supplements important?

Supplements should never take the place of eating well, but a good-quality multivitamin and mineral can be helpful as several factors can affect the nutrients in our diet. Consult your doctor first, as many can interact with certain medications.

Taking vitamin D is non-negotiable, and we should all be taking it every day as we are now so careful about using SPF, which may reduce our production of vitamin D through exposure to sunlight. We need vitamin D for strong bones, mental health, and immune function. Most multivitamins and minerals contain a basic dose of 400IU, although I suggest 1000IU daily for midlife women as a maintenance dose.

There are lots of
ways that the right
nutrition can help to
calm your nerves,
boost your mood,
and put the spring
back in your step.

—

GUT HEALTH

This is a hot topic right now, and understanding the impact of the "gut microbiome" on overall health is vital. The microbiome is the bacteria and other microorganisms in the gut, which help to break down food, and there are many factors that can impact the balance of this bacteria. Prioritizing gut health not only supports digestion, but also contributes to a resilient immune system and vitality. In fact, experts now consider the gut to be our second brain, because of how much influence it has over both our mental and physical health.

Q & A
Sophie Medlin, Dietitian, Director of CityDietitians, and Chair for the British Dietetic Association, London

How do we know if our gut is functioning as it should?

If you're going for at least one poo a day and you're not getting bloating or wind that troubles you, your gas and stool isn't particularly smelly, and you're not getting stomach aches, then you can assume that your gut function is pretty good.

The key to understanding gut health is the microbiome. The trillions of organisms that make up the gut microbiome are like a beautiful habitat, the bacteria and other microorganisms all working together.

How does our diet impact the gut microbiome?

What we eat affects which microorganisms thrive and which don't. When our diet is plant heavy we can benefit from the amazing compounds they produce: we call these postbiotics, and they help to regulate inflammation, support brain health, and control appetite. Gut health is about looking after those microbes, but it's also about looking to your gut function for clues as to what might be going on within your microbiome.

What might we experience when our gut health is not in balance?

Things like poorer immunity, struggling with your mental health, and brain fog can be signs that your gut health perhaps isn't so good, and of course there are clues such as constipation, diarrhoea, wind, and bloating. But these are all what we call bi-directional: poor mental health can be perpetuated by poor gut health, but it can also impact gut health.

Are there any other symptoms that are actually rooted in gut health?

We now think that almost everything roots back into the gut, and there are loads of reasons to look at your gut health if you're having any symptoms at all.

Symptoms Linked to Gut Health

- **Skin reactions:** the gut–skin axis is currently a heavily researched area
- **Sensory issues:** temperature fluctuations and dizziness can be due to increased sensitivity to histamines in food in midlife
- **Mental health concerns:** including brain fog, anxiety, and depression
- **Sleep problems:** the sleep hormone melatonin interacts with gut bacteria

Does gut health affect our brain?

The gut and brain are hormonally connected by the HPA axis (which affects metabolism and mood), and physically connected via the vagus nerve (the main part of the nervous system). When you're anxious, you're more likely to be bloated, constipated, or have diarrhoea: all signs that the gut and brain are connected.

Approximately 95% of the body's serotonin is housed in the gut, and while we're yet to understand how that directly connects to our brain, sharing such a key neurotransmitter in both organs is a sign of a strong connection. Our gut microbes also produce GABA, a calming hormone, and dopamine, a happy hormone.

How do our hormones impact gut health during midlife?

We notice gut microbiome changes after the menopause, and we don't know whether that's directly linked to the hormones or whether it's the stress of the menopause. A lot of my midlife patients say they used to be able to eat whatever they wanted, but now their gut seems much more sensitive. We think this is because of the reduction in diversity of bacteria that occurs during and after the menopause.

One recent discovery is a particular species of bacteria that helps to harvest or recycle oestrogen in the body so it can be absorbed back into the bloodstream. This research is not ready for clinical practice, but is an example of interesting and important things that are going on.

What food is best for our gut?

If you're having debilitating gut symptoms, please see a registered dietitian. If your gut function maybe isn't perfect, but you don't think you need medical input, look at adding things into your diet rather than taking things away. Try to make sure you're having 30 different plants a week. People think this sounds terrifying and impossible, but it's just about variety.

Is there anything other than diet that can improve gut health?

Your gut bacteria love when you drink water, and they love it when you move your body. That's not to say that you need to go to the gym every day or endure exercise that you hate, because that then raises cortisol levels, and stress hormones negatively impact gut health. It's about finding movement that works for you, that feels good for your body, and that you can sustain.

What should we be avoiding?

The gut doesn't like ultra-processed foods. Midlife is a stressful time, and during times of high pressure we often lean on more processed foods for convenience. I see patients who have heard that fruit has got

Dietary Variety

- Add blueberries and raspberries to your morning porridge, maybe some chia seeds and a few nuts: before you know it, you've got five or six different plants just in your breakfast.

- Herbs and spices also count towards your 30 plants per week, and are key to ensuring all varieties of gut bacteria are being fed and can ferment and release their important compounds.

- Include plenty of wholegrains, increasing fibre intake gradually to give your gut a chance to adapt; aim for 30 grams a day (the UK national average is 15).

too much sugar, so they don't eat it and snack on processed protein bars instead. It's far better to choose things like apple and peanut butter or carrot sticks and hummus as a snack. Our guts also don't like alcohol very much, and there's a perfect storm that can happen in midlife where women may increase their alcohol intake due to increased stress.

How about coffee and tea?

Coffee and tea contain anti-inflammatory compounds and polyphenols, a bit like antioxidants, which our gut bacteria actually really like. It's about how much we're having, and whether they are displacing other things in our diet.

What should we be wary of? And is there anything else you'd recommend?

Wherever there's public interest, there will be people ready to exploit that. Steer clear of anything along the lines of gut cleanses, colonic brooms, or colonic irrigation: we really want to look after those bugs, not disrupt them.

There's lots of interest in fermented foods, which produce bacteria that feed our oral microbiome, oesophageal microbiome, and microbiomes in our rapid digestive system. Unfortunately, most of the microbes from fermented foods are unlikely to get through to the colon alive, so if you want to improve your gut health, it is important to feed the bugs that you've got already and perhaps consider a probiotic product.

Probiotics are live, beneficial bacteria that have been shown to support our health. Supplements should be viewed as the icing on the cake rather than a substitute for an optimum diet. There are also prebiotics, which are food for the good bacteria, and these can come from eating a varied diet with plenty of plants.

What about other supplements?

The gut, like any other organ in our body, is influenced by nutritional deficiencies, and when it's not functioning effectively it can cause nutritional deficiencies. Ensuring you're getting enough B vitamins, iron, omega-3, and vitamin D is important for

Probiotics & Prebiotics

- Probiotics can be found in fermented foods like kefir, and in capsules, liquids, and powders.
- There are "smart" probiotics available, containing bacterial strains that may help reduce cholesterol, cortisol, and stress hormones.
- Always choose delayed-release capsules, because otherwise the bacteria will get killed off by stomach acid.
- Foods containing prebiotic fibre include artichokes, onions, garlic, oats, bananas, and nuts.
- Prebiotics also come in functional foods like fibre bars, capsules, and powders, and are sometimes included in probiotic capsules.
- If you have digestive symptoms like bloating or gas, avoid supplemental prebiotics until those symptoms have resolved as they can make them worse.

healthy gut function. This can be through your diet or in supplement form, but remember that certain types of iron in supplement form can cause constipation. Multivitamin supplements can be helpful, but I'd encourage people not to go to some of the big high street supplement companies because they'll sell you armfuls of stuff and you can end up taking too many. If you do want tailored advice on supplements, see a dietitian.

Fitness

In my almost 40-year quest to keep fit and control my weight, I think I have pretty much tried every exercise regime – some with great success, others less so – from step aerobics, swimming, tennis, and Zumba to Pilates, yoga, running, and kick boxing. But my problem was, even if I did find the time to do it, I would get bored quickly. And I know there are many women who have never really liked or done much exercise at all, variously not having the time, money, or confidence to start.

EXERCISE IN MIDLIFE

Some women in their 40s and beyond might avoid exercise due to injuries. I experienced my first bout of sciatica after deciding to take up running at the age of 40; the constant pounding on the pavement caused a slipped disc, with shooting pain radiating down my right leg. I was sent to a sports rehab specialist, who advised me to leave behind high-impact exercise programmes and instead focus on building up my core strength and muscle mass with gentler, yet just as effective, exercise regimes such as yoga, Pilates, or strength training.

EXPERT ADVICE
KATE OAKLEY, YOUR FUTURE FIT

We can lose as much as 3–8% of muscle mass per decade after 30, and this appears to accelerate with naturally declining testosterone once we hit perimenopause, affecting our strength, power, balance, posture, and aerobic capacity.

Additionally, oestrogen starts to decline, which is the key hormone for protecting and maintaining bone density, and bone starts to break down faster than it's repairing. We can then become susceptible to osteoporosis, with one in two women facing a fracture over the age of 50.[1]

Our body's ability to deal with stress can impact how we exercise during midlife. Declining progesterone reduces the body's ability to buffer our stress hormone, cortisol, and low oestrogen affects our ability to cope with the subsequent stress on the body. Exercise that our bodies once tolerated or even thrived on, such as high intensity interval workouts (Hiit) or long cardio sessions, can, for some, cause too much stress on an already stressed body, exacerbating feelings of fatigue, and may not necessarily be the answer to weight management.

It's important to reassess how we exercise in midlife. This chapter brings together experts who specialize in three restorative low-impact regimes: strength and resistance training, yoga, and Pilates. These are incredibly helpful in relieving some of the mental and physical symptoms of the menopause. There are many other low-impact and aerobic regimes that we can all easily adopt and enjoy, such as walking or swimming. Experiment with what works for you and find something that you enjoy so it becomes part of your routine rather than a chore.

STRENGTH AND RESISTANCE TRAINING

This is about far more than getting beautiful biceps, although that's always a nice bonus. It is predominantly concerned with building back up muscle mass, which we start to lose fairly rapidly in midlife, and keeping our bones strong to protect from developing bone fractures caused by osteoporosis. It's also important to build core strength and protect the spine so we can cope with everyday tasks and stresses that require power, strength, and balance, such as lifting bags and bending over.

Q & A
Kate Oakley, Personal Trainer
and Founder of YourFutureFit

What is the best way to work out in midlife?

I set up YourFutureFit because I'd learnt first-hand how exercise can be part of the solution when menopausal symptoms impact our lives. Not only can it improve the quality of our lives now, but it also serves to future proof our bodies as we focus on building our strength, fitness, and healthy habits.

One of the most important forms of exercise to prioritize in this life stage is resistance training. I would then add to that some weekly cardio for heart health and ideally some yoga or Pilates to work on agility, flexibility, and balance.

What is resistance training?

It is a form of physical activity that requires you to move a muscle or muscle group against an external resistance: this can be dumbbells, your own body weight, resistance bands, weights machines, even bottles of water; any object that causes the muscles to contract. As the muscle contracts, it tugs and pushes the bone,

Resistance Training Benefits

- **Increases muscle mass:** essential for everyday weight-bearing tasks such as lifting
- **Improves bone health:** reduces chance of injury later in life as bones will be able to bounce back
- **Enhances mental wellbeing:** serotonin and endorphins produced when you train are antidepressant biochemicals
- **Increases energy levels:** renews your ability to deal with life's challenges
- **Reduces vasomotor symptoms:** helps with menopausal hot flushes, night sweats, and migraines

which stimulates bone growth. As your muscles become stronger, the harder they pull, meaning your bones are likely to become stronger too.

And the best news? It doesn't have to take place in a gym, involve lots of expensive equipment, nor mean hour-long workouts several times a week. Resistance training can easily and effectively be done in your own home or garden, or even when out for a walk.

What's an easy way to start?

While you're brushing your teeth you can do a few bodyweight squats, or try a wall squat: press your lower back against the wall, as if you're sitting on an imaginary chair, and hold for as many seconds as you can. This will primarily work the front of your thighs (quads). If you use this time to strengthen your body twice a day, that's 28 minutes a week – a full workout that you didn't have to find any extra time for. All these little things do add up: think about how many times in the last month you've thought, "I've only got 10 minutes, so it's not worth bothering with." Multiply that across the month. If that's seven or eight times, you're heading towards an hour and a half of potential exercise, so those 10 minutes are absolutely worth doing. Some simple exercises include:

- press ups against the sofa for chest, shoulders, and abs
- triceps dips off the sofa for arms
- bodyweight lunges as you walk around
- getting out of a chair without holding onto the arms, to build leg strength
- walking up the stairs or escalator

Are you ever too old to use weights, and how heavy should they be?

It is never too late, whether you're in your 60s, 70s, or beyond. Weight depends on your starting point; it's best to be assessed by a personal trainer, but as an average starting point I suggest a pair of 3kg for the upper body and a pair of 4kg or 5kg for the lower body.

YOGA

The first time I tried yoga was when I was pregnant with my eldest child, as a good friend had told me it may help with the birth. It was incredibly relaxing, and I couldn't believe I hadn't tried it sooner, but guess I always thought it was reserved for those "ballerina" types who were already perfectly toned and flexible, certainly not for someone like me.

In more recent years I've discovered how helpful yoga can be for midlife women, with it being widely advised that activities such as yoga may help manage the mood swings and anxiety experienced during perimenopause and menopause, as well as help with symptoms such as hot flushes, night sweats, and insomnia.

Q & A
Petra Coveney, Founder of Menopause Yoga

How can yoga help women in midlife?

The menopause is a biological, psychological, and cultural transition. It affects the whole person – mind, body, and emotions – so you need a holistic approach. Yoga is a uniquely holistic practice designed to help manage physical conditions and find mental balance. It includes movement and poses (*asana*), breathwork (*pranayama*), and meditation (*dhyana*), as well as hand positions (*mudra*) and affirmations (*mantra*).

However, yoga is not a magic pill on its own: it complements other medical, healthcare, and lifestyle support. And not all styles of yoga are beneficial for some menopause symptoms: for example, hot yoga can trigger hot flushes and headaches, dynamic yoga such as Ashtanga could exacerbate joint and muscle pain, and certain breathing might trigger anxiety or panic attacks. I have curated a series of menopause yoga classes tailored to help specific symptoms and navigate this time of change.

What is menopause yoga?

It provides practical tools and techniques that may alleviate symptoms, a positive framework to help you embrace change, and a sense of community so you're not alone on your journey. It includes practices for things like menopausal rage and irritability, designed to soothe and calm, as well as practices to relieve anxiety, brain fog, headaches, migraines, fatigue, hot flushes, and digestive issues.

How can we fit yoga into our lives?

Try to do a little every morning and evening, and write down what you did and how you felt. Finding time for a 15–20-minute practice can make a huge difference to your day. However, if all you have time for in the morning is a five-minute stretch and two minutes of breathing, then later in the day you can try to fit in a couple of yoga poses. Doing some gentle stretches next to your bed at night tells your body and your brain that you are preparing for sleep.

How do we get started?

You can begin with something as simple as a menopause restorative pose followed by *Savasana*, which is the corpse pose for relaxation. This is always the final posture in any yoga sequence, where you lie flat on your back with eyes closed and consciously relax every part of your body.

This posture helps to increase energy levels, reduce insomnia, improve mood, increase blood flow, stimulate digestion, and relax the entire nervous system.

Can yoga help to alleviate troubling symptoms such as hot flushes?

Hot flushes can be triggered by both environmental changes and by the food and drink we consume, but also by stressful thoughts; and it can be a vicious circle if we feel embarrassed when we have a hot flush, because the stress makes us feel hotter. The key is to relax into the sensation and use some simple tools to help you feel more in control. You can practise the breathing techniques shown on the following page anywhere.

Yoga Benefits

- **Regulates the nervous system:** helps to reduce mental stress
- **Releases physical tension:** this improves sleep and digestion
- **Improves flexibility and reduces pain:** stretches and strengthens muscles
- **Mobilizes joints:** improves mobility, especially after injury
- **Develops balance:** helps prevent falling that may lead to fractures
- **Improves mental health:** alleviates anxiety, overwhelm, and low mood

Breathing Techniques

COOLING STRAW BREATH

- Purse your lips and suck air in slowly as if sipping a cold drink through a straw, and pause at the top of your inhalation.
- Slowly exhale out of your nose so that the exhale is longer than your inhale.
- Repeat for 3 sets of 10 reps, and then breathe naturally.

COOLING SMILING BREATH

- Smile and breathe air in through the sides of your mouth, pausing at the top of your inhalation.
- Slowly exhale out of your nose so that the exhale is longer than your inhale.
- Repeat for 3 sets of 10 reps, and then breathe naturally.

OCEAN BREATH

- Lay on your back with knees bent and feet on the floor, placing one hand below your belly button and one hand at your lower ribs.
- Breathe into the space under your hands and notice the movement of breath flowing in and out like a gentle wave.
- Inhale through your nose, and slowly exhale out of your mouth, making a soft whispering sound at the back of your throat.
- Repeat for 3 sets of 10 breaths.

Could yoga help with menopausal rage and irritability?

"Menorage" is like another form of heat in the body, a surge of hot emotion that rises up suddenly and explodes. The original cause of your emotion may be justified, but the sudden escalation into anger might be damaging to relationships. You need to channel that energy and release it positively in a way that feels more in control. Create some space between you and the situation, and try the following.

- **Candle breathing with birthday cake visualization:** breathe slowly in through your nose, pause at the top of your inhalation, then purse your lips and softly breathe out of your mouth as if you were blowing out candles. The exhalation should be longer than your inhalation. Repeat for 3 sets of 10 breaths. Every time you exhale, you've blown out more candles so by the end there is only one left and your breath is very gentle. Celebrate and smile.
- **Hand mudra and mantra:** open the palms. Inhale slowly through your nose, and as you exhale touch the tip of your first finger to the tip of your thumb and slowly whisper "Saaaaaaaa". Inhale, touch thumb to middle finger tip and exhale "Taaaaaaa". Inhale, touch thumb to ring finger and exhale "Naaaaaa". Inhale, touch thumb to little finger and exhale "Maaaa". The exhalation is always slow and longer than the inhalation. Repeat three times.

Can certain yoga poses help with any digestive symptoms?

Yoga cannot change the cause of digestive symptoms, but the following poses may help to alleviate them:

- **Legs raised restorative pose:** lay on your back, raising your legs up on a chair and resting your hands on your abdomen, and breathe into the space under your hands. Inhale through your nose, and as you exhale sigh out any tension. This will relax your jaw, which relaxes your diaphragm and tells your body to rest and digest.
- **Windscreen wiper twists:** lay down on your mat, bend your knees, and place both feet flat, about hip distance or wider apart. Inhale through the nose, then exhale out of your mouth (ocean breath) and gently lower your knees to the right side, rolling onto the outside edges of your feet. Inhale and bring your knees back to the centre, hug knees to the chest, then exhale and lower knees gently to left side. Repeat four times on each side. Twists can help with the release of gas and elimination of waste.

Is yoga also good for pelvic health?

We can use pelvic floor exercises with breathing techniques to tone the pelvic floor area. This increases the pleasure of penetrative sex because you are toning those muscles that become weaker as the oestrogen declines around the vaginal wall area. Yoga also assists with bladder control, with exercises to reduce the risk of waking up at night needing to pee.

How does yoga help to protect our bones during menopause?

Yoga cannot build bone density to prevent osteoporosis, but all poses that stretch the muscles and ligaments may benefit bone health. The following poses will help with balance, and build muscle mass and tone to support the whole skeletal structure. They can all be practised with a wall or chair for support, and should be held for 60 seconds.

- **Tree pose:** stand on one leg and bend the other knee, turn your knee outward to stretch into your hip, and place the sole of the foot either inside your other thigh or at your ankle (but never near your kneecap).
- **Warrior 3:** balance on one leg and lean forward with your other leg raised up behind you in a T-shape.
- **Half-moon pose:** balance on one leg with your chest turned to the side and your arms open.

Osteoporosis is often associated with kyphosis, which is the rounding of the upper back. There are some yoga positions that can help to prevent this spinal deterioration by toning the muscles along your back, and these include Cobra lifts and Locust poses.

EXPERT ADVICE
LOUISE MINCHIN, TV PRESENTER, AUTHOR, AND ENDURANCE ATHLETE

To those who say it is too late to start a new sport or hobby, I would argue that is not true, it is never too late, and until you try you won't know what you are capable of. For me, the benefits of taking on big challenges later in my life have been huge. It has changed me both physically and mentally, and I am stronger and fitter at 55 than I was a decade ago.

- **Start slowly:** no one runs a marathon on their first day. When I first started triathlon, I could hardly run any distance at all. Couch to 5k app is one of the best ways I know to start running from scratch. It builds you up very slowly, only running a minute at a time at the beginning, and within a few weeks you find yourself running for half an hour.

- **Form a habit:** consistency is key, so try and make exercise part of your life. Put it in your diary along with everything else you need to do. Join a class that you commit to going to every week.

- **Make it non-negotiable:** if you are part of a team you are going to need to turn up for them, there is no option. Sometimes I get myself dropped off far from home so I have no choice but to run or cycle back.

- **Call a friend:** one of the most powerful motivators is to find a friend who will keep you company

in your chosen sport or hobby, and who will also keep you accountable.

- **Have a goal:** I find that setting a challenge is incredibly helpful. I am always more motivated when I'm training for something specific, otherwise the grind can feel relentless. Your goals don't have to be big goals: they are yours, so choose them wisely. Make them big enough to stretch you, but not so big that they put you off.

- **Find your tribe:** look for a club that will support you. It could be online or in person: look on Facebook and more than likely there will be a beginner's running club near you, or a group of walkers, a road cycling club, a gang of open-water swimmers, a triathlon club, a Zumba class. My experience of mostly everyone who has joined a club is that they are there because they are passionate about what they do and will be delighted to help you.

PILATES

My personal favourite exercise regime, when it comes to movement, toning, and looking after my posture and pelvic floor health, is Pilates. My daughter introduced me to it as she has long been a convert, and it only took about four sessions before I was totally hooked too. I was amazed by how I managed to keep up with her, and at how quickly I was able to build up my own core strength.

For the first time in my life I have found an exercise that I genuinely look forward to doing. Pilates gives me body confidence and provides me with an hour where I totally switch off from thinking about anything else. I now do it religiously three to four times a week.

"

For my 50th birthday, I decided I wanted to get really fit. I'd never had any time for myself while I was bringing up a family and working full time, and I just didn't like feeling constantly lethargic and out of breath every time I walked out the door. I had also become a lot flabbier around the belly.

I started going to a Pilates class twice a week, and noticed such a difference in my core strength and stamina within about a month. I am the fittest I've ever been, and my body is so much more toned, flexible, and healthy looking. It feels so good to be fit in midlife. If I can do it, anyone can!

SHIRLEY, 50

Q & A
Dinah Siman, Menopause Pilates Founder

What is Pilates?

It's a very logical and in many ways intuitive conditioning system. You learn a lot about how your body works, and it focuses on strength, balance, bone loading, mobility, and flexibility. Some movements in Pilates are similar to yoga, with one of the main differences being that Pilates has a lifestyle philosophy rather than a spiritual practice. Pilates is known for working on the core, and as a method of exercise it's appropriate for anybody: you can use it from rehab all the way up to elite sports level.

Pilates Benefits

- **Builds core strength and mobility:** this is achieved in a supportive way
- **Strengthens muscles and ligaments:** this helps to support joints
- **Targets areas precisely:** uses focused resistance work
- **Adaptability:** every exercise can be tailored to your needs
- **Helps with weight management:** just 15–20 minutes a day of strength Pilates helps to speed up metabolism
- **Cardio health:** low-impact exercise benefits heart, bones, and muscles

How can Pilates help women in midlife?

Pilates is a very safe method of exercise. Many midlife women feel too tired, sore, or experience symptoms such as frozen shoulder or plantar fasciitis (inflammation of the foot), which stop them moving. Add to that the weight fluctuations that often occur in midlife, and many women don't want to go to the gym or be in big classes. Pilates is the perfect way back in to movement, a safe technique that meets the needs of the midlife body. Resistance can be added to make it more challenging, and all exercises can be modified for any individual injuries or issues.

Can it help with pelvic floor health?

All Pilates classes have a focus on breathwork, by teaching lateral breathing and ensuring the diaphragm is moving. Because of this breathwork and the focus on core muscles, Pilates can be really beneficial for the pelvic floor. However, if someone has pelvic floor issues it's important that they are seen by a women's health physio, so we know where we're starting from, because often women need their pelvic floor to be released as much as strengthened. And there is a lot of retraining required if you have got incontinence or bladder issues. Taking time to lie down and quietly observe how your body moves naturally is a great way to start connecting with your pelvic floor.

How often should we do Pilates?

You could do it on a daily basis, or you could do it a couple of times a week, it's about what works for you. You could focus in one session on strength and upper body work, and then have another session later in the week which is more about relaxation, calming the whole system down, and releasing joints.

Can we do it at home?

A lot depends on experience, but once you understand the basics, home practice is key. Fit short exercises into your daily routine, like Sit to Stand, a functional movement where you are sitting and standing from a chair – a great way to get in what I call a "movement snack". Recent reports[2] discuss how beneficial isometric exercise (contracting muscles while the body is held in one position) is, particularly for blood pressure. Do simple isometric moves, like a wall squat, during the day.

Is it hard to commit to a Pilates routine?

It can be challenging, and there are many reasons in the menopause transition that make us want to stop exercising. If you know that you struggle to commit, then I recommend you book in advance for,

Pelvic Floor Exercise

- Lie down and bend your knees, feet flat on the floor hip-width apart. Your gaze should be up or slightly forwards.
- Place your hands each side of your rib cage and focus on your inhalation and your exhalation. Inhale through the nose and gently exhale through your mouth. Notice how your ribcage opens as you inhale and drops back down as you exhale. Stay with this awareness for 4–6 breath cycles, then relax.
- Place one hand on your lower belly and one on your ribs, and repeat the breathing practice. Again notice how your body expands and relaxes.
- You can feel your abdominal wall and ribs moving. The diaphragm contracts down the body as we inhale, and the pelvic floor is mirroring this.

say, a six-week course, or team up with a friend to encourage each other.

If you are new to Pilates, definitely have a chat with your teacher first. It's really important to communicate, and if you've got specific needs, such as injuries or problems relating to menopause, then they need to be aware of that. If you want to be sure that a class is for you, ask to go and watch first to get a feel for it. If you've already been practising for a long time, keep going, don't stop, because Pilates is an exercise method that will see you right the way through to your old age.

Sleep

Sleep issues can be debilitating during midlife and menopause. Lots of women complain about disrupted sleep and its devastating effect on their ability to function at work and home, as well as on their relationships. Both men and women face challenges that may be affecting their sleep, however, there are some that are unique to women, such as hormone fluctuations, maternal stress, menstrual cycle changes, and menopausal hot flushes. So it's not at all surprising that women in their 40s and beyond can have multiple factors that give rise to significant sleep disruption.

SLEEP ISSUES IN MIDLIFE

While some women cope well with less sleep, for others it can have a massive effect on their daily lives, impacting physiological processes, causing productivity and energy levels to plummet, and putting them at an increased risk of other health problems. Cognition and memory can also be massively impaired.

One of the worst symptoms I experienced during perimenopause was insomnia, surviving on three hours sleep a night if I was lucky. Trying to work on so little sleep became almost impossible, and was one of the main reasons why I had to quit my job during that time. And I've heard similar reports from numerous women within The Latte Lounge community.

66

I am 45 years old and have suddenly developed insomnia. I go to bed at roughly the same time every night, but I struggle to fall asleep, and even when I do I usually end up waking up three or four times in the night and can lie awake for an hour or so. It is so frustrating. I have tried so many different things, but nothing is helping and I'm absolutely exhausted. It's making it increasingly difficult to hold down a job, and is also affecting my marriage.

MATILDA, 45

Q & A
Professor Guy Leschziner, Consultant
Neurologist specializing in sleep disorders

How common is insomnia among midlife women?

Insomnia is incredibly common, with about 30% of adults experiencing it in a year. Insomnia is more common in women than men, and a recent study shows that insomnia may affect as many as 60% of perimenopausal and menopausal women.[3]

What helps govern how we sleep?

There are two biological mechanisms that physically influence our sleep. The first are the circadian rhythms, your own internal body clock, driven by a small area in the centre of the brain. Your body clock defines the times of the day you feel sleepy and feel awake. Most people tend to want to go to sleep somewhere between 10pm and midnight, and wake up between 6 and 8am, and there is also a natural increase in sleepiness in the early afternoon.

The second is the homeostatic mechanism, which means that the longer you have been awake, the more you want to sleep. In simple terms, this is driven by certain chemicals within the brain that build up over the course of wakefulness and then reduce once we're asleep.

What are the effects of our changing hormones on our ability to sleep?

The sleep cycle is greatly affected by hormones, and many women who are still menstruating report a difference in sleep quality in the latter half of their cycle, where sleep is more fragmented. There is also an impact on sleep quality and quantity caused by the fluctuation in hormones during perimenopause and menopause, and due to symptoms such as hot flushes, which are incredibly disruptive to sleep.

Other problems can occur around the time of the menopause because of changes in fat deposition and distribution. Women may gain weight, or the areas of the body where fat is deposited

may alter, resulting in changes in the chest region and the neck, contributing to a condition called obstructive sleep apnoea. This affects individuals who snore, where they develop a partial or complete obstruction of their airway, and this tends to increase dramatically around perimenopause.

How can we help ourselves?

We need to step back and prioritize ourselves, and begin by incorporating some basic habits for good sleep hygiene. Sleep hygiene is simply getting into habits that promote good-quality sleep. It's important to say that good sleep hygiene is not going to be the difference between somebody who's got chronic insomnia and somebody who is a good sleeper, but if you have intermittent poor-quality sleep, then changing some of your behaviour surrounding sleep is important.

Insomnia may affect as many as 60% of perimenopausal and menopausal women.

Good Sleep Hygiene

- **Cut back on caffeine** as it can hang around in your bloodstream for up to 8 hours. Avoid after lunch, replace with decaf, a herbal drink, or water.
- **Don't use electronic gadgets after 9pm** as the blue light impacts our internal body clock, taking over the production of melatonin (the sleep hormone) and making it difficult to drift off. Put your phone or tablet down at 9pm and leave them in another room when you go to bed.
- **Avoid alerting activities** such as engaging with social media or watching a movie late at night.
- **De-stress** by taking 15 minutes before you go to bed to stop and move away from the build-up of the day's mental stress.
- **Have regular bedtimes:** go to bed and wake up at a regular time. The brain is a creature of habit when it comes to sleep, so regularity is beneficial.
- **Reset the sleep/bed association:** don't go to bed when you're not tired as it increases the subconscious association between bed and being awake. You need to reset the brain's association between bed and sleep (this is the basis of CBT for sleep problems).
- **Watch what you eat:** regulate the time that you eat your last meal, and avoid eating large, carbohydrate-heavy meals late at night.

Can exercise and diet help us to sleep?

We know that exercise, particularly aerobic exercise, is good for promoting deep sleep – what we term slow-wave sleep. We would generally recommend not vigorously exercising in the last couple of hours before sleep though.

You'll come across a lot of dietary supplements that claim to boost melatonin levels or promote certain chemicals within the brain, but the evidence for that is limited. The key thing is to avoid large meals in the hour or two before bedtime: a very full stomach might contribute to abdominal symptoms and predispose you to reflux at night, and rich meals may cause disturbances to your blood sugar overnight and defragment sleep.

What are the reasons behind persistent poor sleep?

There are a number of changes that occur in chronic insomnia, some psychological and some physiological and biological.

PSYCHOLOGICAL FACTORS

Some psychological factors are conscious. A lot of people will experience significant anxiety or frustration at the prospect of either trying to go to sleep or being unable to sleep, with fears about whether or not they're going to be able to function the following day and about lying awake. There are also fears about what the lack of sleep is doing to their long-term health, which in many cases are unfounded. There are also a lot of unconscious factors. For most of us bed is a place of comfort, which we associate with having a good night's sleep. But in individuals with chronic insomnia, their bed is associated with being awake and struggling to get to sleep.

One of the fundamental treatments for chronic insomnia is to try and reprogramme the association between bed and sleep, which is when CBT for insomnia (CBTi) really comes to the fore.

BIOLOGICAL FACTORS

Biological changes occur when you've had poor sleep for a prolonged period. Levels of adrenaline, the major hormone and neurotransmitter involved in the fight-or-flight response, go up, so people can feel exhausted, wired, and jittery as they enter into this state of hyperarousal.

We also know that the stress response hormone cortisol is very good at inducing insomnia. Cortisol also goes up when we've had very poor-quality sleep, so you can end up in a vicious cycle whereby the psychological factors drive poor sleep, then biological factors cause it to get worse.

How does CBTi help?

Cognitive behavioural therapy helps to rid people of the anxiety related to insomnia and uses the brain's own mechanisms that drive sleep to rebuild positive associations.

CBT for insomnia is becoming the gold standard treatment because it works very well for the vast majority of individuals. It is not the only psychological treatment available, but we know that 60–80% of individuals have shown a significant improvement in their sleep with CBTi alone.

What kind of medical treatment options are available?

In previous decades, the first thing that a doctor would reach for is a prescription for drugs like zopiclone, zolpidem, and benzodiazepines. But we now know that these medications don't simulate normal sleep. They're sedatives rather than sleep promoters. And there are issues associated with these drugs being addictive or dependency forming, with people requiring long-term, ever-increasing doses.

There are alternatives that are perhaps less likely to cause dependency, and I do use some of those drugs in individuals who are particularly resistant to other forms of treatment, but they are not the first choice. In the last 20 years or so there's been a sea change in how we address insomnia, and I strongly countenance the move towards a non-drug-based approach such as CBTi as the first-line treatment for insomnia.

60–80% of individuals have shown a significant improvement in their sleep with CBTi alone.

—

Can HRT help with sleep?

HRT is a very evidence-based solution for poor-quality sleep during perimenopause and menopause. It's helpful in restoring hormone levels to a point where they're not disrupting sleep quality. In the past the usual pharmacological treatment for the perimenopause was SSRI antidepressants, but given that HRT will address sleep issues as well as the other perimenopausal symptoms, it has become a first-line pharmacological treatment in this setting. For those who are unable or choose not to take HRT, CBTi and other non-pharmaceutical approaches are commonly recommended.

Many midlife women complain of "Restless Leg Syndrome" affecting their sleep. What is this?

It's a neurological disorder that causes an urge to move typically your legs, but it can affect other parts of the body. That urge is often associated with an unpleasant sensation and aching, tingling, cramping, or some other form of discomfort, and tends to come on at night. RLS is often worse when we are tired or relatively sleep deprived, so it may be that during perimenopause and menopause, when our sleep is getting worse anyway, it might bring the RLS to the fore. There is anecdotal evidence that oral magnesium supplements or baths with Epsom salts can provide some relief from RLS.

What does the future of sleep therapy look like?

A major development has really been an evidence base for non-drug-based therapies. There have been a few drugs that have either come to market or are coming, but for the vast majority of people, drug-based treatment is not necessarily where they should be going.

But for those of us who are just bad sleepers, rather than classed as insomniacs, it's important to recognize that this is usually just a blip. Sleep is innate. Don't label yourself as a "bad sleeper" as there is so much you can do to help, and everyone has the ability to get a good night's sleep.

EXPERT ADVICE
MARYANNE TAYLOR, FOUNDER OF THE SLEEP WORKS

CREATE A SLEEP ROUTINE

- **Reflect:** take 5 minutes to write down the positives you experienced in your day and jot down tomorrow's to-do list.

- **Review:** spend a few minutes processing and reviewing your to-do list. Put a deadline by each action, then set it aside.

- **Relax:** raise your body temperature with a warm bath or shower. The drop in body temperature afterwards helps stimulate the production of melatonin (known as the "sleep hormone").

- **Stop, look, and listen:** STOP: calm your racing thoughts with some deep-breathing exercises. LOOK: read a book, or try mindful colouring to help you wind down. LISTEN: enjoy relaxing music, a podcast, or an audio book.

- **Ignore the clock:** don't stare at the clock and calculate how many hours of sleep you have left. This only increases anxiety. Turn the clock around and let go of the time. If you can't sleep after around 10–15 minutes, get up, relax in a different space, then return to bed when you feel sleepy.

- **Temperature control:** ensure your bedroom is kept at around 18°C (64°F). If you are suffering with hot flushes and night sweats, lightweight, breathable clothing and good-quality bed linen can help. Keep the room as dark as possible.

- **Avoid heavy meals:** heavy, spicy meals in the evening can affect metabolism and cause discomfort, making it more difficult to fall asleep.

- **Hydrate:** drink plenty of water during the day, but limit liquid intake from late afternoon to avoid nighttime bathroom trips.

- **Final tip:** incorporate a simple breathing technique when you get into bed to facilitate a calmer body and mind, preparing you for a restful night's sleep.

Restoring Calm

The perimenopause and menopause years, combined with the pressures of looking after ageing parents and often still having caring responsibilities for children if we have them, can have a significant impact on our mental health. How can we take back some control and feel less stressed? While some women may want or need to explore medication and therapy, many experts now recommend that we try incorporating practices such as mindfulness, meditation, and hypnotherapy into our lives.

MINDFULNESS AND MEDITATION

One of the problems of midlife is that we don't know how to adapt to all this change. We seem to be getting busier all the time, doing things faster than ever to keep up, and this causes us to get stressed and feel like we can't stop, even for a second, to catch our breath. This is where mindfulness and meditation can change everything.

These practices may initially sound a bit "woo-woo", but when you understand what they entail and learn how to incorporate them into your day, they can transform the way you cope with life's pressures and help with some of the more troubling symptoms of the perimenopause and menopause. As always, when looking for a therapist, make sure they are registered with an organization accredited by the Professional Standards Authority (see p.248), and ideally have a healthcare background.

Q & A
Natasha Nicole Harris,
Mindfulness and Wellbeing Coach

What is mindfulness?

It's the act of bringing our attention to what we are doing right now in this very moment, rather than letting our minds wander off to the past or the future. When we are not mindful we get swept along and are not fully engaged, so things just happen to us, and often not in the way we want. But when we bring our full focus and attention to the present moment, we give ourselves choices and have an opportunity to powerfully change the way things play out.

Is it hard to do?

I often hear that people are hesitant about mindfulness because they find it difficult to meditate; many believe that meditation is about sitting in a yoga lotus pose for 30 minutes or longer without moving. So when my clients come to me and tell me they find it nearly impossible to sit for even 10 minutes and switch off their minds, I get it. While you can be mindful while you meditate, you certainly don't have to meditate to be mindful.

How do mindfulness and meditation differ in practice?

Mindfulness allows us to become more conscious of our thoughts and our inner dialogue: are we speaking to ourselves in a kind and compassionate tone, or are we harsh and critical? As you start to notice these subtleties you will bring about a wonderful awareness. Without awareness, we cannot change anything and continue to feel powerless.

There are many techniques that help us to quieten the mind and become more in tune with the present moment. We can become more mindful while brushing our teeth, doing the laundry, or on a walk out in nature. Meditation though, is still usually about sitting quietly and putting time aside for this practice.

How can we practise mindfulness?

You can make a start by being fully engaged in this moment. The next time you are having a conversation, notice where your attention goes. Does your mind wander off? Or are you focusing on everything the other person is saying? Are you aware of what's going on around you? The people, the noises, the smells? How are you feeling? Every passing moment provides an opportunity to be mindful. Mindfulness is not something we "do", but it is more a state of being. You can practise mindfulness:

- for just 10 seconds
- while chatting with a friend and still actively listening
- when walking down the street and noticing everything around you
- while focusing on your breath
- while reading this book
- you *are* practising mindfulness when you notice that you need to stop and take a break

Mindfulness Benefits

- **Better attention span and focus:** you are more efficient because you're not easily distracted
- **Feeling calmer:** because you are not trying to do too many things at once
- **Body and mind can rest:** enjoy a break from the endless background chatter
- **You experience flow:** things slow down, but you can still get things done
- **Relationships improve:** both with others, and with yourself
- **De-stress:** you can let go of day-to-day stresses and anxiety
- **Fewer conflicts and more balance:** a calmer mindset impacts your actions

What happens when I forget and get caught up in the busyness of life?

Don't worry, this is part of the process. The second you realize that your mind has become distracted, you are being mindful. Simply remind yourself to come back to the present moment. It's a cycle: we are mindful; we get distracted; we realize we are distracted; we become mindful again.

Over time, I have become quicker at noticing when I'm being mindful and when I'm not. I'm less anxious about what I can't control and approach things with a calmer attitude, I have better sleep, and I enjoy better relationships than I have ever had before.

Any other advice on being mindful?

We're all different, and what works well for one person might not work at all for someone else. Find what works for you, and keep practising it. And be patient: it takes a little time for things to become our new "normal". It's often said that we need to try things out for 21 days to establish new patterns of behaviour. Practise little and often: doing something for 20 seconds a few times a day is better than not doing it at all.

How can we take our mindful practice a step further and begin to meditate?

Once you've created awareness, you can develop this practice in your quiet space. I always say start small: put aside five minutes, go into a quiet space, and turn off your devices. Focus on your breath: your in-breath, and your out-breath. Really be curious about it. Is it short and sharp, or long and deep. Are you breathing into your upper chest, or into your belly? Does it feel uncomfortable at any point? What is happening to your shoulders? Pay attention to what's happening, and if it begins to change.

Just two minutes is enough to begin with, and doing this two or three times a day is far more beneficial that trying (unsuccessfully) to sit still for 10 minutes. If you start to do it as you wake up every morning, your whole day will start to feel different.

What are the benefits of meditation versus simply being mindful?

Meditation is a wonderful way to slow down and be still. We are all so busy running around and "doing", always switched "on", our nervous systems on high alert. When we give ourselves permission to actually stop, even for a few minutes, things really do change. As we start to practise meditation, we can feel calmer and more centred, and our perception of the outer world also slows down. It's a beautiful thing to be able to create for ourselves in such a busy world.

Simple Mindfulness Exercise

- Walk down the road today and try to really notice everything
- Put your phone and any other distractions away
- Notice the people passing by: what are they wearing? Are they smiling, or serious?
- What cars are on the road?
- What are the buildings like on the opposite side?
- What have you walked past 100 times before and never noticed?
- What else do you notice?

HYPNOTHERAPY

What first comes to mind when you hear the word "hypnotherapy"? Relaxation, a deep sleep, or perhaps being taken into a trance-like state? Hypnotherapy can sometimes be misunderstood, but for many women it can be a lifeline, significantly helping them with their symptoms of perimenopause and menopause.

Hypnotherapy can help to reduce stress and ease symptoms such as hot flushes, anxiety, and sleep disturbances, and it can even support women with more general health anxiety too.

Q & A
Sally Garozzo, Clinical Hypnotherapist

What is hypnotherapy?

It's based on the science of neuroplasticity, and I believe it's a viable treatment option for the mental health challenges that arise during midlife. Hypnotherapy takes advantage of the hypnotic state, during which people can be more open, receptive, and highly suggestible. In order for lasting change to occur, it's important to access feelings rather than just logical thought. During hypnosis we are less inhibited, so feelings and emotions tend to pop to the surface without resistance, and we can leverage these to help make powerful decisions and lasting changes.

What is happening within the body and brain during a hypnotherapy session?

During hypnosis there is a change in brain activity. EEG scans have shown an increase in theta brain waves, which are slower and linked with relaxation and focused attention. fMRI scans have shown that the hypnotic state can indeed shift perceptions, enabling a different way of processing information, especially to do with physical and emotional pain. In a 2016 study published in the *Oxford Academic Journal*,[4] scientists attempted to discover what physical changes were occurring in the brain under hypnosis.

Hypnotherapy Benefits

- **Helps get to the root of problems:** can assist with getting to the bottom of psychological issues quickly
- **Positively reframes attitudes:** this can be attitudes to food, exercise, alcohol, and relationships
- **Help to change the way we think:** resulting in more calm, inner peace, and resilience
- **Allows us to navigate change:** helps us to make shifts in our identity and core values to better support our changing circumstances
- **Helps us set better boundaries:** in both our work and personal lives
- **Self-care:** we are more awake to our own needs, and increase our self-care

They discovered that there was reduced activity in the part of the brain responsible for executive function, planning, cognitive flexibility (task switching), and inhibition.

With all this in mind, hypnosis can be a useful state to carry out therapeutic interventions, allowing us to get to the crux of the issue quicker without having to wade through layers of "masking".

How is hypnotherapy particularly beneficial for women during midlife?

Hypnotherapy is especially useful to help with the mental and emotional turmoil that can arise at midlife and menopause. It's also very good at helping to reframe how we experience our symptoms. By rapidly rewiring the neural pathways in our brain using powerful suggestions, we can down-regulate our fear response and even alter our perception of physical sensations in the body.

Is hypnosis something you can do alongside other medical treatments?

Yes, it slots in perfectly with treatments like HRT, acupuncture, aromatherapy, and counselling. In order to know if hypnotherapy will benefit you, some therapists will do a suggestibility test during the consultation and others will send you a pre-session recording to discover how easily you can access the theta state. If you feel you're drawn to hypnotherapy, the likelihood is that it's something worth investigating.

Can people get some of these benefits at home?

You can get some benefits from hypnosis recordings on YouTube or Spotify. These provide a boost of energy and bathe your mind in positive suggestions that can leave you feeling calmer or more confident. However, working with a therapist gives maximum impact because they will be able to guide you through a powerful process and help you to see those exiled parts of yourself more clearly.

Self-Care

The hormonal and age-related changes associated with midlife and the menopause give rise to a whole host of confidence-knocking concerns, from body-image issues to worries about our skin and changes in hair quantity and quality. As well as taking care of our health and learning to relax, there's never been a more important time to stop and think about the way we care for ourselves on the outside too, addressing struggles with self-confidence.

HAIR CHANGES IN MIDLIFE

Our hair is often an intrinsic part of our identity, and is a key indicator of our health and wellbeing. A great many women experience hair loss (alopecia) and hair thinning during midlife and menopause, which can have a huge impact on self-esteem. There are myriad reasons for this, including hormones, genetics, nutrition, and certain medical conditions.

I've personally noticed a huge amount of hair thinning around my temple area, and it really does affect my confidence. I've tried numerous different lotions and potions to counteract it, mostly to no avail. And I know I'm far from alone, having heard from hundreds of women over the years, all looking for solutions to their midlife hair concerns.

> *I've had problems with hair loss most of my adult life, but since the menopause it's been thinning really fast. It's so thin over the top section and starting to recede at the temples. I've tried minoxidil for a year, and Nourkrin, but neither have made any difference. I take multivitamins and iron daily. My doctor has not been particularly helpful, and it's making me so self-conscious.*

ISOBEL, 58

Q & A
Dr Hélène du P. Menagé, Consultant Dermatologist

What are the main hair changes that occur in midlife?

As we age, the hair shaft itself becomes thinner and more follicles go into a resting phase, leading to a reduction in hair density and finer hair. The reasons for this are not fully understood, but are often genetically determined, in the same way that some women can grow their hair longer than others due to the variable length of the anagen phase of the growth cycle, and as we age this cycle shortens. The three phases of the hair growth cycle are: growing (anagen) phase, 2–7 years; transitional (catagen) phase, around 2 weeks; hair falling out (telogen) phase, 3–4 months.

How likely is it that we will actually lose our hair over time?

Women rarely go bald in the same way that men do, unless they have a specific disorder. We don't lose our frontal hairlines but the hair there does get thinner, and most of us will experience a degree of female pattern alopecia as our fluctuating hormone levels have an impact.

How do environmental factors and lifestyle affect the hair?

There's no real evidence that environment affects hair loss and thinning, but lifestyle factors can have an impact and can alter our perception of the problem, particularly stress. Diet also plays a part. If you have a reasonable diet and no malabsorption issues, then you should have no nutritional deficiency. But so many women tend to follow restrictive diets or start to yo-yo diet around menopause, and when we suddenly reduce our carbohydrate load, we push hair into the telogen stage, so 3–4 months later we notice significant hair loss.

There are also some medications that can damage our hair. We are familiar with hair loss with chemotherapy, but other treatments such as retinoids, anti-clotting agents, certain hormones, other cancer drugs, and occasionally lipid-lowering medications can also be associated with hair loss.

What should we do if we are concerned about our hair loss?

For women suffering with alopecia, it's important to see a doctor; you don't necessarily need to see a specialist, although this can be useful in some cases to have the scalp checked with dermatoscopic examination to rule out any possible underlying condition.

Trichologists (specialists in hair and scalp problems) are not doctors, but they can be helpful, particularly in situations when access to primary care and dermatology is limited. Doctors can check for nutritional or thyroid deficiencies, and may consider testing for autoimmune conditions and other hormonal conditions if clinically indicated.

Your doctor may wish you to check in with a dermatologist. It is advisable to take any test results and medical history with you. Some specialists may repeat certain blood tests and will examine the scalp with a dermatoscope. It may be necessary to send away for a scalp biopsy to look for any scarring and inflammation.

What nutritional deficiencies affect the hair, and can supplements help?

It's important not to get carried away with taking supplements, and to make sure there is sufficient evidence for your requirements before you take them. Some common nutritional deficiencies and therapies are listed below.

- Iron deficiency can affect your hair, so iron tablets will be recommended. These should be taken with vitamin C to help absorption.
- Low vitamin D has been linked to hair loss, as has zinc. The minimum recommended vitamin D supplement for everyone is 400IU between October and March in the UK, but many will

need more and require it all year around. This can be determined with a blood test.

- Biotin (one of the B vitamins) has been hailed as helpful, but may interfere with troponin, a heart blood test.

What medical treatments are available to help with hair loss?

It depends on the cause, which is why a proper diagnosis is important. An exciting recent development is a new medication (JAK inhibitors) for autoimmune hair loss, but pattern alopecia remains the most common diagnosis in the perimenopause.

Don't rush out and spend a fortune on treatments, try a holistic approach first which focuses on sleep, a balanced diet (avoiding crash dieting), exercise, mindfulness techniques to reduce stress, and careful hair styling.

Some medications may be used "off-label" to treat alopecia. An off-label medication is one that has not been officially approved by the regulation agency for this particular use. Approval is a long and expensive process, and a drug may not be approved simply because it has been in use before the approval process came into place, or, and this is often the case, because it was found co-incidentally to help a condition.

If treatments fail and the impact on the person is high, then hair pieces, wigs, and transplants are sometimes considered.

Hair Loss Treatments

- **HRT** is not proven to help hair, and hair loss isn't an indication for treatment, but HRT can be helpful in impacting overall mood. However, it is important to be careful about which progesterone you take as this can impact the quality of your hair, too.

- **Vasodilators** such as minoxidil (which improve circulation by widening blood vessels) are known to help and are available without prescription as topical applications. Oral minoxidil may be prescribed off-label. Extra facial hair can be an adverse effect, and gains are lost on discontinuation.

- **Anti-androgens** (which block hormones like testosterone) may help, such as bicalutmide, dutasteride or finasteride, off-label. These are forbidden in pregnancy (usually used for pre-menopausal women). Topical anti-androgens are being trialled, hoping they will have fewer adverse effects than oral administration. Other forms of local delivery such as micro-needling are also being explored.

- **Spironolactone** (a diuretic medication) is now increasingly offered off-label to help with alopecia.

- **Experimental treatments** such as low-level laser and light treatments (LLLT), and "vampire serum", which is plasma-rich protein injected into the scalp – an expensive and not wholly convincing treatment.

HAIRCARE AND STYLING

When it comes to things to do with hair that are more within our control, a good hairdresser can help work miracles. They can offer expert advice on how to best protect, cut, and style hair to deal with issues around greying, thinning, and changes in hair quality, as well as advise on treatment options that will and won't work. By this point in our lives we usually know what suits us and what doesn't, but when it comes to helping our hair to look as good possible in midlife, products, techniques, and styling can make a big difference.

Q & A
Michael Douglas,
Celebrity Hairdresser and Founder of mdlondon

What are the main differences you notice in women's hair in their 40s or 50s, compared to their 20s and 30s?

Some women's hair gets thicker, more coarse, dry, and brittle, while others becomes thinner and finer. Hair thinning is normal as you age, but if you are worried about the amount of hair you are losing, it's best to talk to a trichologist, an endocrinologist, or a dermatologist. Cells replicate the cell that came before, so as you get older the previous cell is slightly more deteriorated than it was. So it is inevitable that your hair will ultimately show signs of ageing: the big question is, how confident do you feel about how old you look and how old you are, and what steps are you prepared to take in order to address that? There are a lot of things we can do to alleviate certain concerns, it's a case of how much time have you got and how much do you care about it?

Do thickening shampoos or other such styling products work?

Shampoo cleans your hair; that's what it's supposed to do. If you start expecting it to do loads of other things, you're ultimately going to be disappointed. Simply use a shampoo that best suits your hair type – particularly if it's highlighted, bleached, or coloured – and which you feel is working for you.

Volume, body, and thickness comes in the styling stage, and are largely about technique, using a blow-dryer with a decent nozzle and a smallish bristle brush along with styling product. Resin-based products like mousse and blow-dry spray are good for adding in volume.

The key ingredient to look out for is PVP/VA copolymer, a setting agent that hardens onto the hair; it can go crispy, but if the hair is kept moving during drying the crispy feeling disappears and you are left with hold and volume. Generally stay away from any oil-based products such as serum and hair oils as they are heavy and create zero volume.

Can you recommend any particular cuts that create body?

It's not easy to generalize, and different face shapes really don't matter, so don't get tied up in all of that.

People ask if layers will make hair look thicker and fuller, but what layers do is take away from the internal bit of hair, so we lose all the thickness at the ends. Layering can often make hair look thinner and wispier if you've got fine hair. With a bobbed hair style it's all the same length at the bottom, so you can get a real sense of fullness, brilliant if you've got fine hair.

Is it easy to use extensions and hair pieces to help hair look thick or fuller?

Some simple hair wefts can help fix a whole bunch of concerns. They're perhaps not for everyday wear, more a confidence boost for a party or big work presentation.

- **Clip extensions:** at the back of your head, hair grows all the way from crown to nape, but at the side it only grows half the distance because of your ear, so it's always thin from here because there's half the amount of hair. Putting in two clip extensions on the left and right-hand side just above the ear fills this area out.
- **Double-weft clip-in hair extensions:** a weft is a piece of material with hair sewn onto it, and double-wefts are two of these stuck together, so you get a nice, thick bunch of hair. They're not massively expensive, depending on the length and the colour you want, and come in different sizes. Clip these into your own hair, combing them in and thinning them out a bit at the ends, and they will make such a difference to hair that's looking a bit thin and flat.

How can we transition from colouring our hair to embracing grey?

Most people want to disguise the line between the natural hair growing through at the root and the coloured hair on the mid-length and ends. The temptation is to colour some of the roots to break up the line, but it's hard to disguise that line unless you're covering 70–80% of the roots with lowlights or something to match the ends. But then you'll be growing out the highlighted bits endlessly. So my advice really is to grin and bear it, and just grow it. A year will give you 12–14 cm (around 5–6 in) of growth, so just keep on cutting the colour out until it's gone.

Is grey hair coarser and drier, or is it the same as if it still had colour?

I think it can feel that way. The cortex (surface layer of the hair) is what houses all of the colour pigments, and when you stop producing those colour pigments, the cortex changes a little bit.

But lots of people who have gone grey have hair that feels silky and soft. It really is different for everyone. If your hair is feeling thirsty and dry, treat it to a really good conditioning treatment like Coconut Miracle Oil. All the supermarkets sell it, and it is the best thing I've used. Put it on your hair for 10–15 minutes a week, or every five shampoos. The active agents in the oil attach themselves to the surface of your hair like a fake cuticle that's much smoother than the one you've got.

Can dyed hair still be healthy? And should it only be done at a salon?

Most of the box dyes in the supermarket use the same chemical compounds and the same science as you get in the salon. Don't

be fooled into thinking that because it's on a supermarket shelf it's somehow much worse for your hair, as the process is exactly the same. The main difference you get from the salon is somebody to choose the colour for you and to apply it.

If you're just colouring grey hair there's really little to worry about regarding the effect it has; the way colour works is by opening the cuticle scales at the surface of the hair, the colour seeps into the cortex, swells up, and gets locked inside. So every time you colour your hair, you open the cuticle layers a tiny bit. This is arguably what is called "damage" to the hair, but you'd have to open the cuticles a lot to cause much damage. So if you are colouring your hair with a permanent colour every 6–8 weeks, it's really nothing to worry about.

Is it OK to continue to lighten our hair as we get older?

The more you lighten your hair, the more significant damage you're causing, because you're essentially decomposing the inside of the hair. If you've got a mixture of blonde hair and grey hair and you're putting bleach on it and lightening it a lot, if you weighed a strand of the hair it would probably weigh about two-thirds less than before it was bleached. So bleached blonde hair is very damaged, highlighted hair is less so, and the least damage is caused when you dye the hair a shade darker.

SKINCARE

Over the last decade I've noticed a massive difference in my skin. Where it was once bright and glowy, even though in places spot prone and oily, it is now much duller, dryer, and itchier, and it feels like my jowls are drooping by the minute. There are masses of midlife women who are looking for solutions to everything from sun-damaged skin and wrinkles to rosacea, dermatitis, moles, skin tags, and acne, all of which are affecting their self-confidence. Happily, there is plenty we can do to help improve our skin's appearance in midlife, during menopause, and beyond.

Q & A
Dr Amiee Vyas, Practitioner in Aesthetic Medicine and Founder of Doctor Amiee Facial Aesthetics & Skin

Why do our faces show signs of ageing as soon as we hit midlife?

Up to this point, oestrogen has been our skin's best friend. It has been boosting hydration, helping to keep skin plump, encouraging the production of collagen, controlling oil glands, and keeping our skin clear of breakouts. As we enter perimenopause, we start to lose oestrogen and the skin becomes dry.

Also, as we age, the bone structure of the face changes. Our cheek bones become flatter and the fat pads that sit on top of them lose volume and start sagging due to the lack of bony support. We lose volume in the mid-face and gain volume in the lower face, causing lines from the nose to the mouth (nasolabial folds), then "marionette lines" (wrinkles at the corners of the mouth), and eventually jowls. Loss of collagen and elastin are accelerated by age and menopause; this impacts the neck and décolletage, where the skin becomes loose and wrinkly. And we must never underestimate the cumulative effects of an unhealthy lifestyle, which compounds all of the above.

Lifestyle Factors

- **Get a good night's sleep:** sleep is often negatively impacted in menopause, resulting in increased cortisol, which can worsen or trigger inflammatory skin conditions.
- **Hydrate well:** drink 2 litres (3.5 pints) of water every day to keep skin hydrated and mitigate the harmful effects of a pro-inflammatory lifestyle (one high in sugar, salt, alcohol, and processed foods, and includes smoking).
- **Top up on antioxidants:** your diet should be rich in multicoloured fruit and veg to boost antioxidant capacity. Skin can become more sensitive in midlife, and antioxidants can help to repair the skin barrier.
- **Avoid excessive sugar:** too much sugar causes a skin-damaging process called glycation, which is accelerated during the menopause. Skin relies on the scaffolding of strong structural collagen; excess sugar causes collagen fibres to become weak and rigid, resulting in wrinkles and a dull complexion.

What are common complaints you see in your clinic from midlife women?

Women tell me their skin is incredibly dry, and their wrinkles and lines feel like they appeared almost overnight. This happens as our collagen significantly depletes (by 30%) during the first five years of menopause, and you can feel totally unprepared. Next comes jowling, and the feeling of looking tired and sad. This is because of bone changes and volume loss in the cheeks, which also reduce support under the eyes.

Can our ethnicity affect the extent of skin changes?

Age-related skin changes are certainly different depending on ethnicity. My patients with darker skin tones will complain of dehydration, texture, and pigment concerns before complaining of wrinkles and sagging. This is because darker skin already lacks ceramides, which help lock in moisture, at baseline compared to white skin, and the skin structure in darker skin tones is more robust, so wrinkles and sagging tend to present later than in white skin.

Women of colour's skin has more melanin (pigment) at baseline, and this is distributed widely through the skin structure compared to Caucasian women's skin. Hyperpigmentation is therefore the main concern for darker skin tones, while lighter skin tones are more likely to notice age spots related to high sun exposure.

Do you think collagen drinks and supplements actually work?

While these are popular at the moment, overall I don't believe there is enough evidence at present to support their skin benefits over a healthy diet and lifestyle.

Collagen significantly depletes (by 30%) during the first five years of menopause, and you can feel totally unprepared.

—

Daily Skincare Routine

- Use a gentle hydrating cleanser in the morning and evening.
- Follow with a moisturizer: look for ingredients like hyaluronic acid and ceramides.
- For the daytime, finish with a minimum of SPF 30 all year round.
- In the evening use a retinol before moisturizer: start at the lowest strength and apply sparingly if you have never used one before as they can be drying.

What non-invasive treatments are there?

I am an advocate of medical grade and prescription-strength skincare, which works beneath the surface of the skin, down to the dermis, where collagen and elastin is produced and which contains the matrix that keeps skin full and plump.

- Start with skincare that's professionally tailored for your skin type.
- Chemical peels are ideal for those who are worried about downtime and want to avoid injectables. Controlled ingredients like acids and retinols/retinoids stimulate collagen and elastin.
- Radiofrequency and lasers work by stimulating the skin's structural proteins and resurface the skin.
- Micro-needling induces a mild injury in order to trigger collagen production and enables better penetration of active skincare ingredients.

Starting some of these treatments early, in our 30s and 40s, improves skin quality so that when we reach the stage where our hormones change, we don't see such a rapid decline, and we can even prevent a lot of the changes.

What is the next stage, if women want to step up their treatments?

The next stage is minimally invasive injectables, which make a profound difference and really impact patients' confidence. The term "injectables" encompasses treatments that are injected into the skin and facial tissues. This includes botulinum toxin (commonly known by the brand name Botox), dermal fillers, skin boosters, biostimulators like Profhilo®, and polynucleotides which improve how skin cells are functioning at all levels.

Are injectables a last resort treatment?

There are preventative ways in which we can use injectable treatments like botulinum toxin and dermal fillers. People always get the wrong idea about these treatments, but when used in the right way, with a full-face approach, using minimal amounts, you can actually prevent the descent of tissues. If we start to do this just as patients begin to notice the changes, we can mitigate those effects from happening in the future. It's essential that you see an experienced

Injectable Treatments

- **Botulinum toxin** is used to temporarily paralyze muscles to minimize the appearance of wrinkles that happen as a result of repeated expressions, such as frown lines, forehead lines, and crow's feet. It can also be used to treat a downturned mouth and counteract the pull of strong lower face muscles, which can alter our appearance with age. Botulinum toxin is also used for purely medical applications including treating migraines and teeth grinding.

- **Dermal fillers** come in many varieties, but the most popular are hyaluronic acid gels, which can be used to correct or enhance volume loss and structural changes; they can also be used to rehydrate. Hyaluronic acid fillers are reversible, but other dermal fillers composed of polycaprolactone as well as other ingredients are non-reversible and provide longer lasting results.

- **Skin boosters** also come in many varieties: they may be hyaluronic acid-based, such as Profhilo®, include specific vitamins and minerals, or be composed of ingredients such as polynucleotides, which all work to improve skin cell functioning and therefore improve skin quality. Profhilo® is recommended as a course of two treatments, which are repeated once or twice a year, depending on your age. Polynucleotides require a course of two–three treatments done once or twice a year depending on your age, skin quality, and skin concern.

medical professional for injectable treatments. They will be able to tailor a treatment plan to give you the most natural, long-lasting, and beneficial results for your skin type. They will also be able to advise you when *not* to treat.

What treatments offer the longest lasting results?

In order for treatments to last longer it is vital that you combine them with the right skincare. Botulinum toxin is a prescription-only injection and lasts three-to-six months, but if you use it with the right skincare, and repeat your treatment within the appropriate time frame, you will prevent deep, embedded expression lines from forming. Over time, the gaps between treatments lengthen. I have patients that I've seen for years who now only have treatments once or twice a year.

Dermal fillers will last around a year. Again, these are best done in combination with skincare, or with radiofrequency or lasers. Medical practitioners have access to premium medical-grade injectable products that are safer to use and last longer. Be aware that there are many unregulated non-medical people offering these treatments: not only do they lack the skills to administer these treatments properly, they also won't have access to premium, safe, and effective products. Always ask for their credentials and the details of the products they are using.

MAKEUP

In midlife, many women lose confidence and don't like how they look in the mirror anymore. Yet something as simple as reviving your makeup routine can make a huge difference. Women can feel stuck in a rut, still using the same techniques and products as in their teens and 20s. But often what worked then doesn't seem to look quite so good on midlife skin. I certainly have a lot to learn when it comes to perfecting application, but you don't have to have the skills of a professional MUA to enjoy the feelgood effects of makeup.

Q & A
Ruby Hammer MBE, Makeup Artist

What part does makeup play in building our self-confidence?

Tailoring products to your specific needs allows you to enhance the elements you love and camouflage the ones you don't. Get comfortable with your own reflection, looking into a mirror and reacquainting yourself with your features. Concentrate on what is in front of you *now*, don't lament what you once had. Wrinkles aren't the element that let down your face, they show you have lived, it is the tone and pigmentation: an even skin tone looks radiant and healthy.

How can we discover what will best suit us, and learn to apply it correctly?

Many midlife women will have figured out a personal skincare or makeup routine over the years, and will be experts in what products may or may not have helped. But as we approach the perimenopause and menopause years, the skincare and makeup routines we have become used to may need to be tweaked, especially if you are experiencing hot flushes or maybe have noticed that your skin has become dryer and perhaps a little duller than it used to be.

Knowing how to apply makeup is really just about practising until you become confident. You will know after a few attempts if you have blended it enough and whether it suits you. You will soon see if an eyeliner looks better on the waterline or on the outside of your eyelids. It's often personal preference.

Do you have any application tips for when we want a full face of makeup?

With cosmetics there are two golden rules: like goes on to like, and *blend*. Cream products can be applied easily over other cream products, and powders applied over powder products. When changing textures (from cream to powder), set with a thin veil of translucent powder to avoid streaking and uneven application.

It doesn't matter how many products or in what order you apply them as long as you blend, blend, blend! With bronzer, if it's powder, prep with a translucent powder beforehand to avoid streaks. With blusher, apply to the apple of the cheeks and work upwards and outwards, not getting too close to the eyes for an everyday radiant look.

What are some common makeup mistakes, and how can we rectify them?

The most common mistakes I see are usually around using too much makeup, when in fact we need to use makeup more sparingly as we age, avoiding being

Making Up Midlife Skin

- If you are prone to hot flushes, set foundation or eyeshadow with powder to avoid it sliding off.
- Apply thin layers of foundation, or it could look cakey and sink into any lines, making them appear more visible.
- Select a good concealer in two different weights – one lighter and more fluid for around the eyes, and one a little thicker for skin concerns like rosacea or blemishes.
- Brush loose translucent powder lightly over areas where you want to blot shine and set areas where you've applied concealer.
- Invest in a few good brushes and a magnifying mirror.
- Curl your lashes with an eyelash curler, and wear a good mascara.

too heavy handed with everything. And again, it's important to remember to blend well, especially under the chin and along and down the neck, so that it all looks tonal and uniform.

If you have hooded eyes, try losing the eyeshadow and concentrate instead on a bit of tightlining on your eyes. But there really is no magic wand, no right or wrong way to apply, so have fun experimenting. And you don't need very expensive products either, there are some lovely brands out there in every price bracket.

PERSONAL STYLE

When it comes to self-confidence, it's not just about
skincare and makeup but also about being confident
in how we dress for the next chapter of our lives.
Approaching midlife can feel daunting, perhaps bringing
insecurities to the surface and with them a loss of
confidence and identity. Our changing bodies and worries
about what's "appropriate" for our age play a part, and we
are constantly bombarded with messages about body
confidence online, and quite often faced with ageism in
the fashion industry. Upheavals like returning to work
after a career break, or leaving the workforce after many
years, can create their own wardrobe crisis, too.

*I'm returning to work next week after eight years off with my three young
children, but I have no clue what to wear anymore. I used to work in an
accountancy firm where everyone wore suits, but my friends tell me
people are a lot more relaxed in what they wear these days to the
office. Also, I'm plus size. How do plus-size ladies look tidy and
professional? I always feel I look messily thrown together.*

GEMMA, 41

But it really doesn't have to be daunting. By finding a
style and choosing colours and fabrics that flatter and suit
our individual tastes along with our changing bodies and
lifestyles, we can learn how to adjust or even create an
entirely new look to feel cool and confident at any age.

Q & A
Gayle Rinkoff, Fashion and Celebrity Stylist

Why do we lose confidence in how to dress at this stage in our lives?

Women's bodies have gone through many changes by the time we get to our 40s or 50s. You may have had children, and will most likely have been through or are currently going through perimenopause or menopause, and with that brings huge body changes.

So what you used to see reflected back at you in the changing room mirror in your 20s and 30s looks completely different when you fast forward 10 or 20 years. Even for those of you who may be slim and haven't gained any weight, it's highly unlikely that your body will look like it did 10 or 15 years ago. And I'm sure that we all have areas that we prefer to keep covered up.

Is it just body changes that have an impact on our style confidence?

There are many factors. For instance, many women that have left the workplace can feel they have lost their "uniform". It's so easy when you are working to think, okay this is my work wardrobe, then not have to think about it, so dressing becomes second nature. But if they are no longer working, many people become unsure of what to wear.

How important do you think fashion and style are in our lives?

They hugely affect our self-confidence. What someone is wearing is often the first thing you notice when you walk into a room, often before you've even said hello to the person. The clothes that we wear reflect (and affect) our personality, behaviour, mood, and attitude. Loads of people work from home now, but our mindset and style still needs to be in a slightly more "working environment" mode. If we're in tracksuit bottoms or leggings all the time, we are potentially not going to perform at our best because our mindset is in relaxation mode.

How can we be more body confident?

Try to stand in front of the mirror and tell yourself what you love about what you're seeing, because everybody is always too quick to criticize themselves. We need to find ourselves again and embrace midlife, experiment and have fun with colour and new styles, which can totally transform the way we feel and look. Don't be afraid to try things that you may never have considered before.

Social media, for all its faults, also has benefits in being able to find people and accounts that you can relate to. Find a few that you feel comfortable following for inspiration on how to wear certain styles or colours and how to put an outfit together. Take some screengrabs, create a little folder in your phone, and have your favourite images to hand when you go out shopping.

How can we feel more confident about wearing more colour?

Colour is a very personal choice. Some people will never wear black as it doesn't suit them or it completely drains their skin tone, but for others it works for them. If black or beige are your thing but you're thinking about wearing more colours, then do it with an accessory. Add a bright pop of colour in a bag, or, if you're feeling braver, a vibrant coat. Even if you love colour, I wouldn't necessarily advise going head-to-toe in one colour.

How can we go about de-cluttering and updating our wardrobes?

It's good to do a wardrobe detox maybe once or twice a year. Set aside a day, pull everything out of your wardrobe, and try it all on. Enlist your most honest friend to help, and tell them not to hold back. Also ask yourself if any of the clothes you currently have could work well in the styling inspiration you saw on Instagram.

My rule of thumb is that if you haven't worn something for two years, then it's time to say goodbye. Create a pile for charity and a pile for resale – many online platforms can help you with that. Sell unloved clothes and invest the funds in something that's better quality, which you will wear for longer. As we get older and experience symptoms like hot flushes and night sweats, we might want to think more about the quality of our clothes: I always recommend wearing natural fabrics rather than polyester.

Do you have any advice on buying new clothes?

We should all spend some time really looking at what we already have, because we live in a very consumer-driven society where we are told we've got to buy this or have that, and quite often we really don't.

Try to stand in front of the mirror and tell yourself what you love about what you're seeing.

You've probably got something in your wardrobe that will already do the job. When you do want to splurge on something new, there are some great brands that have finally managed to hone in on what grown-up women want to wear to look chic, fashionable, sophisticated, classic, and stylish, with pieces that'll last for years. Amazing tailoring can make all the difference, but these pieces can be a little pricey.

Is it better to shop in person rather than online?

It's good to go to a shop in person to try things on and feel the fabrics, but it can be time-consuming traipsing around large shopping centres. There are loads of little high-street boutiques selling independent brands that are worth exploring, and it's always nice to support the smaller businesses who will quite often give you a much better customer experience, too.

Shopping online is convenient if you're sure on sizing, but it's helpful to edit the overwhelming choice down using filters, whether it's size or style.

Feelgood Styling

- **Draw focus:** anyone can wear anything, but some tricks can help with emphasizing/de-emphasizing features. V-necks tend to flatter a larger bust as it draws the eye to the point of the V; prints work well on smaller boobs; if your best asset is your waist, add a belt to cinch it in, or wear a waisted dress.
- **Wear one colour:** this will elongate you if you'd like the illusion of added height and don't want to wear heels.
- **Be cool:** stick to 100% natural breathable fabrics if you are prone to hot flushes, and think about layering. You don't want to feel like you're having to strip off in public, but removing a layer or two is fine.
- **Clever camouflage:** a scarf is always a great way to camouflage chest wrinkles if you are worried about wearing a high neck top and getting too hot. A scarf can add colour, or dress jewellery can help to fill the space if you prefer an open neck top but don't want to show a big expanse of flesh.
- **Accessorize:** this can transform the simplest outfit, so experiment.
- **Put on your favourite outfit:** even if you're just going to the supermarket, don't always pull on leggings simply because they're the easiest thing. And don't save things for best: if you feel amazing in something, just wear it.
- **Get inspired:** have your favourite style inspiration images to hand when you go out shopping.

SELF-CONFIDENCE

So many women, myself included, have spent years being overly critical of ourselves. And yet, if we were to ask our friends and family to write down all of our amazing qualities, I bet there would be a very long list handed back. So how can we learn to see ourselves in the same light as those who love and believe in us do? We can optimize areas of our lives as outlined throughout this chapter, but without learning to love and believe in ourselves, all these other things are just a sticking plaster. There is so much we can do to reshape this significant life phase into something truly positive. How exciting is it to think we could have a completely new and interesting second act to look forward to right now?

Q & A
Michelle Griffith Robinson OLY,
Olympic Athlete and Life Coach

What can cause a loss of self-confidence in midlife?

Many women come to me with low self-esteem and say it's because they're overweight. Others complain of having impostor syndrome in the workplace, or that they have just lost their way. Some still believe comments made in the school playground, or by unhelpful relatives or past partners. Often women tell me that they look at what they presume to be their "confident" friends and say, I wish that I could be like her. But you don't see when someone is struggling, all you see is what they choose to show you.

I do get a lot of midlife women coming to me because the symptoms of perimenopause and menopause are impacting on their confidence. But I want women to realize that midlife can be a time where, actually, you're at the age when you can and should feel more confident in who you are.

How can we begin to regain our confidence in midlife?

By recognizing our strengths and allowing ourselves to feel confident in our own skin. I always recommend starting with positive affirmations: tell yourself the great things about yourself rather than always focusing on whatever is lowering your self-esteem, and write them down; think about how your friends and family would describe all of your amazing attributes to others.

Is it about accepting and loving where you are, or trying to make changes?

It depends. Say you really want to lose weight: first identify why. What's it for? *Who* is it for? If it's just for you, great, but focus on getting fitter and healthier rather than slimmer. Set some targets, go for a 5K walk, or walk with a friend up the hills. You'll get the results you want and feel better about yourself afterwards.

And let's get rid of this size thing. I'm a size 10/12 and was pre-diabetic for five years, but through working on myself and implementing lifestyle changes I have taken myself out of the pre-diabetic zone. I know women who are larger sizes and are fit and healthy. Don't starve yourself or do "Dry January" – start living a moderate lifestyle. Do some form of movement three or four times a week; it doesn't have to be weight training, it could be getting out for a brisk walk with your dog.

How can we find the motivation to exercise?

You don't have to train five days a week. I want women to let go of this perfectionism and stop thinking that they've got to go all-in with exercise or take up a drastic detox. We all have mornings when we just want that extra half an hour in bed, and I've been there. This morning I didn't want to get up; however, today is my non-negotiable training day. I've made myself a priority, and I'm holding myself to account.

- Write down the days that you are going to do something and then make it a priority.
- Ask your partner or a friend for support and allow them to hold you to account if you don't want to go for that 6pm walk because it's raining outside and there are chores to do.
- Focus on forming good, solid habits that are achievable.

Can clothes and makeup play a part in our self-confidence?

Absolutely. Putting on a pop of colour on a rainy day makes you feel automatically better. It's been proven that you feel better with more colour around you, so try to embrace it rather than hiding behind black and beige. A new pair of shoes, a bit of makeup, treating yourself to having your hair and nails done – these are all things that can make us look and feel good.

How can we avoid comparing ourselves to others on social media?

Sometimes we need a reality check, it's not all as it seems. We generally only share our best bits on social media, so people don't know when we're feeling quite tearful or emotional. If somebody's Instagram isn't adding value to your mood or mental health, delete it and move on. Be mindful of what you're looking at: are you just scrolling because you're bored? Is there something else you can be doing? Read a self-care book instead, or listen to an uplifting podcast.

What are the biggest mistakes women make when it comes to self-confidence?

Number one would be not making time for themselves, not making themselves a priority. Many of us are part of that sandwich generation where we've got ageing parents and also children who we're still trying to guide, so sometimes it does become overwhelming. Reach out and let people know. Meet a friend for coffee and ask for support. Self-care doesn't have to cost anything, a phone call, walking, and chatting are all free. Remember, you've got to put the oxygen mask on yourself first before you can help anybody else.

Confidence-Boosting Self-Care

- Offloading often helps, so ring a friend for a really good chat.
- Set boundaries, say no to things you don't want to do and give yourself some space to think.
- Do something that makes you feel good. Maybe have a "home spa" session, prepare a favourite meal, or take a long walk in nature.
- Know your limits, and try to get enough sleep. Good sleep allows you to feel brighter and more able to deal with everyday challenges.
- Write a list of all the things that make you great, and then put it somewhere to read on those days where you're not feeling quite your sharp self.

I want women to realize that midlife can be a time when you can and should feel more confident in who you are.

—

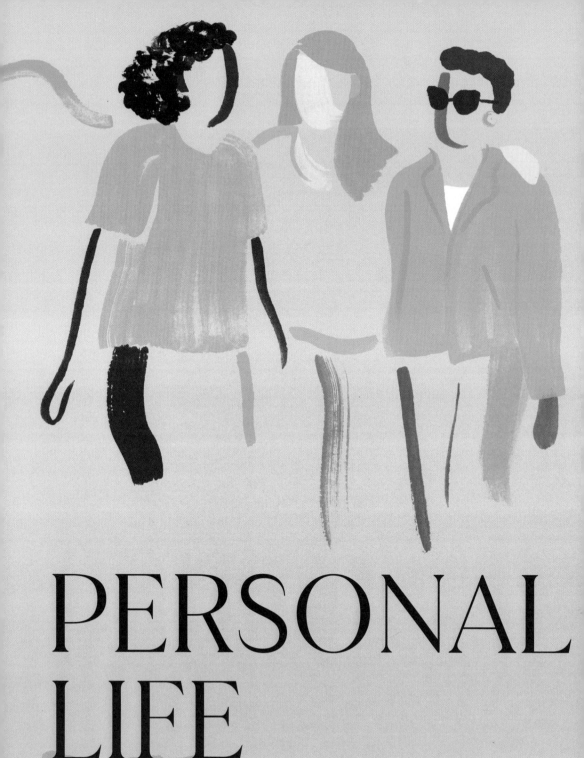

PERSONAL
LIFE

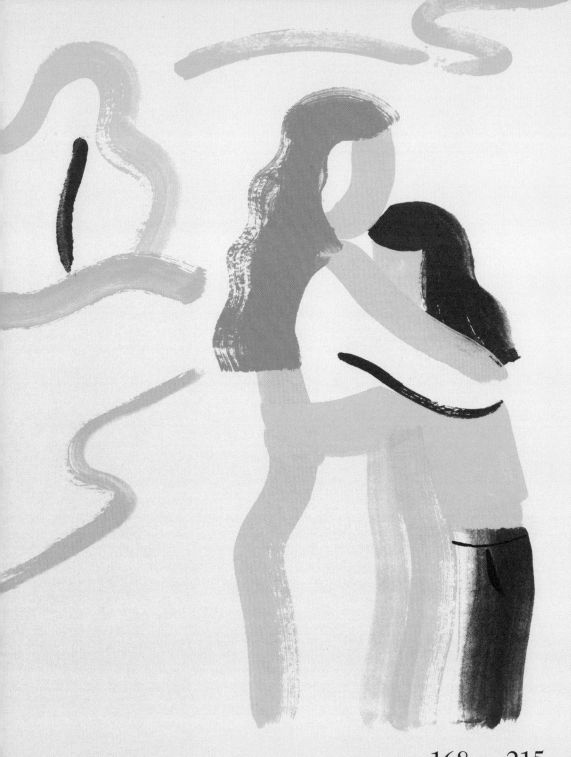

168 — 215

Sex & Relationships

Midlife can offer a sense of liberation, of new beginnings, perhaps with kids flying the nest and maybe a little more financial freedom too, meaning more time to focus on new or existing relationships. But lots of women find they have lost their confidence due to menopausal weight gain, or have no idea how to reignite their flagging libido. And there are those who find themselves newly single in midlife and would like to meet someone but don't know where to begin. As midlife women, there's no reason why we can't have personal lives that are every bit as satisfying as those we experienced in our 20s and 30s.

SEX AND LIBIDO

Enjoying a healthy and fulfilling sex life in midlife is completely achievable with the right mindset and support, especially if we take a more proactive approach and see this time as an opportunity to seize rather than an obstacle to overcome.

When we're dealing with the symptoms of menopause and the stresses of midlife, and particularly if we've been with our partner for a long time, it's not unusual to favour watching a good box set at the end of a long day over anything more amorous. And there's nothing wrong with that, as long as both partners are happy and you are not making yourself feel guilty. As we age, our bodies, confidence, and sexual desires may have changed, and it's important to acknowledge this and educate ourselves about the reasons why libido may be affected during midlife, menopause, and beyond, and understand what we can do to improve things. It's also crucial to keep the lines of communication open and be honest with yourself and your partner.

"

I have zero libido and I just feel like there must be something wrong with me. I've tried supplements, better eating, and exercise, but I just don't want to be intimate. I know it's good for our relationship and I do enjoy it in the moment, but the thought of it and the work up to it, I feel like I just can't be bothered.

I know I shouldn't feel like I have to have sex just to please my husband, but I feel that he needs the intimacy to know that we're okay together, whereas I think most women feel like we need to feel more emotionally connected.

MARIA, 40

If you're looking to regain the excitement in your relationship, or are perhaps in a new relationship and don't know how to get back in the proverbial saddle, there are lots of things that you can do. In the pages that follow you will find ideas for ways you can reignite that fire (if indeed this is something you want to do), learn to love your body, and enjoy a satisfying sex life again.

Q & A
Dr Shahzadi Harper, Author, GP, and Founder
of the Harper Clinic, specializing in women's health

Why do so many women experience a drop in sexual desire in midlife?

Sex during midlife and beyond isn't really talked about. When you think back to when you were in your 20s, if you thought about your parents, aged around 40–65, having sex, you probably would've thought, "urgh, how can they possibly be?" Then suddenly you get to that age yourself and you think, hang on, my life's not over!

Libido is multifactorial. There's no one thing that just switches it off, but we do have biochemical changes going on. Fluctuating hormones from our late 30s and early 40s onwards can play havoc with our sex lives in many ways. Retreating from sex is also your body's coping mechanism: if you're tired you are going to channel your resources and energy into getting through the day, you're hardly going to have any reserves left for sex.

Midlife Factors Affecting Libido

- **Poor sleep:** when you're exhausted, the last thing you want to do is get intimate.
- **Weight gain:** this might cause you to struggle with body confidence and your body image.
- **Poor mood:** many midlife women feel flat in mood, which also affects libido.
- **Drop in oestrogen:** this affects lubrication within the vagina, the thickness and plumpness of the vaginal walls and vulva, and the external genitalia, potentially causing clitoral and/or vaginal atrophy.
- **Declining testosterone:** this can make it harder to achieve an orgasm, or the orgasm isn't as strong as it used to be, which can create doubts and anxiety about the relationship.

What are some of the positives of midlife sex?

The post-menopause years can be a sexually liberating time for women. Those in heterosexual relationships, once their periods have stopped and they don't have to worry about contraception, might feel free to experiment and spice things up in the bedroom. Many may find themselves single again, or perhaps never found "the one", so midlife is a time to reinvent themselves and embrace the women they have become. I hear from so many women who tell me that, regardless of

The post-
menopause years
can be a sexually
liberating time
for women.

—

how they look on the outside, they feel the best they have ever felt in midlife because they finally have time, money, and confidence to spend on themselves.

What is the first step in addressing any problems we might be experiencing?

The first thing to remember is that your body isn't failing you. You still possess that reactive drive, your body can still respond to stimuli, even if you may have lost the initiative to initiate sex. Just knowing this can help. For a lot of women and their partners, it's reassuring to realize that you haven't fallen out of love. But there are lots of things that you can do to improve your libido and sex drive, even though I recognize that it can be difficult to open up that conversation with your partner and/or healthcare professionals.

How vital is good communication?

It's really important, for intimacy, to communicate openly with your partner. You need to be able to reassure them that it's not that you no longer love them, but that at the moment you just don't feel like yourself, your hormones have changed, and explain the impact of that.

It's crucial for your partner to be part of that process to ultimately help you to love yourself and each other more deeply again. Even just going for a walk together and holding hands, or writing it down if you don't know where to start, can make it easier to talk about some of the concerns you may have.

Can men also experience loss of libido and body changes during midlife?

Things do change for men from their early 40s onwards. Their testosterone levels start to decline at a rate of about 2% per year, which accelerates, and although they don't experience depression in the same way that women do, they may become a bit more irritable. The decline in testosterone can mean that they get "dad bods", that pot belly and curvature of the gluteal muscles, and their arms aren't as muscular. Their libido can also drop.

The first thing to remember is that your body isn't failing you. You still possess that reactive drive.

What treatment options are available to help with any physical symptoms?

Women may not even realize that they have got things like vaginal dryness or atrophy because they're not having sex in the first place, but they may be experiencing itching, discomfort, and more frequent UTIs or thrush. These are all symptoms of the drop in oestrogen, which affects the pH balance within your vulva and vagina. There are some really simple things that can be done, which most women have access to (see box, right).

Can testosterone help improve libido?

Testosterone is not necessarily a magic bullet for suddenly reigniting your libido, but it could play a part, and is something that a specialist would prescribe after you've been started on HRT. You do need to have a certain level of oestrogen for it to work well, because testosterone ultimately breaks down to oestrogen. If you've not got enough oestrogen in your body to begin with, then when you use testosterone, it will automatically want to break down to oestrogen to fill your "oestrogen tank".

Testosterone can be prescribed on its own if you do have adequate oestrogen levels during perimenopause. Unfortunately this is still something that many doctors don't feel comfortable about prescribing because there is currently no licensed form of female testosterone within the NHS prescription guidelines.

Treating Physical Symptoms

- **Vaginal oestrogen:** this is available in many different formulations. You can insert a pessary and/or use a cream; the Estring vaginal ring is like an internal moisturizer and can be inserted into the vagina for three months; vaginal capsules such as Intrarosa have some DHEA (the precursor to testosterone and oestrogen), which helps with lubrication and is perfectly safe for women who've had breast cancer. Some brands are available without a prescription.

- **HRT:** (see pp.22–23) can help to improve sleep and reduce symptoms like hot flushes and night sweats, as well as help boost energy, motivation, self-esteem, and confidence – all of which is beneficial when addressing a flagging libido.

- **Pelvic floor exercises:** important to help with strengthening the pelvic floor, because we lose elasticity within the vagina as we age. (See pp.67–68.)

- **Vaginal lubricants:** can also be extremely useful, and should really be used by everyone daily, regardless of whether they are having sex.

- **Sex toys:** can help you to strengthen your pelvic floor muscles because of the contractions, and will also help to improve blood flow.

What lifestyle tweaks can help improve libido?

Even if you feel tired and unmotivated, factoring in some kind of exercise or movement can really boost the happy neurochemicals in the brain. And it helps to tone you by adding muscle, which is so important because we're losing muscle mass due to the changes in hormone levels and the decline in testosterone as well. When we feel toned, it can help us feel more confident in our bodies, which hopefully will help with feeling sexier, too.

It is also important to look at diet and nutrition because we know that the drop in our hormones can impact so many areas, from mental health, which affects body confidence, to the texture of the skin, causing dryness, and even the collagen within the vagina can change. Consuming things like fish oils and making sure you are supplementing with vitamin D can help correct the pH balance in the vagina, and taking a really good probiotic can also help with this.

What about when the problem is more in the mind?

Often there is more to your loss of libido than just the effects of depleting hormones, there's a psychological barrier that's been put up. And for women who've had a hysterectomy or a mastectomy it can feel like they've lost their identity as a woman. This is where psychosexual counselling can be a useful intervention to help you re-establish the connection with yourself and with your partner.

What sorts of things do you recommend in psychosexual counselling?

You don't need to jump straight into couple play, it's about gaining confidence first. To begin with I often talk to my patients about using a sex toy, listening to some erotic apps, or reading erotic books to fire up the neurons in the brain again. When you use a sex toy, you don't have to go full pelt, you can just gently start to press it against your clitoris or nipples to help re-establish that mind–body connection.

I often recommend that you experiment on your own first and then take it into couple play, because when you feel that you can trust your own body, then you will feel more confident with your partner. Even if you don't reach orgasm every time, it's important not to catastrophize and think your body is failing you, and sometimes the journey itself can just be great fun.

Building your relationship back up with your partner should be a priority, too. Discuss not just what you want, but also what you both want, perhaps exploring some of your sexual fantasies together or even just talking about the fact that things aren't what they once were.

DATING

I'm sure there'll be many of you who thought that by the time you'd reached your 40s and beyond, you'd be happily settled with your partner, perhaps married, with any kids getting ready to leave home. But maybe that just never happened, or perhaps it did happen but you find yourself newly single in midlife.

Well, rest assured, you are far from alone, and there are now more single women in their 40s and beyond than there have ever been.[1] While many are happy to remain this way, there are others who'd like a new partner with whom to share the next phase of life. When it comes to dating, the landscape is looking totally different from when we were in our 20s, with apps, websites, gurus, and reams of advice on the dos and don'ts of midlife dating.

When dating in midlife you can draw upon a lifetime of experience, and by now you often know what you are looking for in a relationship, as well as what you don't want. At this stage of your life you may also be more emotionally and financially independent, so are able to invest more time and energy into getting to know a new partner – and maybe having some irresponsible fun along the way!

By now you often know what you are looking for in a relationship, as well as what you don't want.

Midlife dating has been way more successful for me than my younger experience. I had some terrible experiences with women I met online in my 30s – one even brought a panel of ex-partners along to judge if I was appropriate! As a woman in my mid-40s who was more sure of herself, I didn't take any bullshit, and realized I didn't need to go on dates with people who sounded unreliable or flaky. Feeling secure in the knowledge that being single was fine, and that there was less social stigma around it, meant that I felt I had more choices. And it turned out lots of fascinating women were interested. I met my wife online when I was 46, and we've been able to have more mature discussions about what we are looking for in a relationship.

ROSIE, 53

Q & A
Tamsen Fadal, Award-winning Journalist, Menopause
Advocate, and Author of *The New Single*

What are some of the positives of dating in midlife?

The main ones are that in midlife you know who you are, you have the freedom to make your own choices, and you don't feel like you're on some arbitrary timeline anymore. Most of the time, you've either already had your kids and they're grown up, or you decided not to have them, so that conversation's done for the most part. Both people are usually established in their careers, so there's not as much pressure there, and there's so much excitement to look forward to in midlife: the next chapter, next step, next trip, next hobby to do together.

Midlife should be a time for us to take some of the pressure off. Yes, there are ageing parents, there may be kids leaving the nest, and you might have concerns about where you go next: but there is a sense of freedom that comes with it because, quite frankly, it's now or never – this is our time.

There's so much excitement to look forward to in midlife: the next chapter, next step, next trip, next hobby to do together.

—

How do we know if or when we're ready to begin dating again?

Deciding to date again in midlife is basically stepping into a new chapter of your life. It's essential to feel emotionally balanced and content with your own company before jumping into the dating pool. I found that I needed to answer a few questions: what did I want my life to look like? Was I emotionally ready to at least be open to someone to share my life with? Was I more excited than nervous about the prospect of new connections?

It's important to have clear goals – whether you're looking for a serious relationship or just want to meet new people. My goal was not to "find love", but to find new people to share things with. Not all dates worked, but the one that did eventually changed my life.

How is midlife dating different, and what's the best way to get started?

It can be different in many ways; the great part is that we have life experience, but it's scary getting back out there, especially if you've been in a relationship for 10, 15, 20, or 30 years. A lot has changed. Start by refreshing your social skills by doing what you love and are comfortable doing, from cooking classes to outdoor adventures, where you can meet people who share your interests. This helps build your confidence and increases your chances of finding meaningful connections.

With online dating, choose a platform that suits your age and preferences – it's not about the most popular app. And make sure you have a profile that showcases your personality and clearly states what you're looking for in a partner.

Always prioritize safety. Meet in public spaces for initial dates and tell a friend about your plans. And don't feel like it all has to be perfect. Not every date will spark a romance, but each one is a step forward in understanding yourself and what you want in a relationship.

Dating Dos & Don'ts

- **Don't** be afraid of online dating or dating apps: they are not the only way, but they are an option. If you don't know how, get someone to show you.

- **Do** tell family and friends that you are looking to date, because somebody who knows you well could introduce you to somebody else.

- **Don't** go looking for a particular type of person, look for different types of relationships, because along the way you might meet somebody that turns out to be a great friend or confidante, or who may introduce you to somebody they think would suit you better.

- **Do** look for compatibility in important areas. I don't think we have that "perfect person" list anymore, or if we do, we should edit it a little bit.

Dating Red Flags

- **Discussing ex-partners:** be aware if somebody is hung up on an ex and trash talking or relentlessly discussing them. They might not be over them yet.
- **Pushiness:** don't be pushed to go out there and date before you're ready, nor try to convince others to date again before they're ready.
- **Love bombing:** all at once and all too much might sound attractive, but it can be a sign of something you don't want to be a part of long term.
- **Game playing:** be wary of someone who seems too good to be true; not everyone is going to be telling the truth all the time. Have your wits about you.
- **Digital dates:** make sure you meet in person earlier rather than later. If somebody is texting you the whole time and having digital dates but hasn't suggested meeting in person, move on.

How can you regain confidence if you've had a bad experience?

You've got to learn to trust yourself first. It's important to understand the past, but also to move forward and know that it doesn't have to define your future. We often have preconceived notions that, if this happened once, everyone's going to be like that. That's not the case. Looking for consistency in behaviour is key: if you're going to build up your self-confidence and put trust in somebody else, you want to see that they follow through on promises, and not keep giving them excuses if they don't. You've got to set boundaries of what's acceptable behaviour in a new relationship.

Is it better to date our own age group?

I don't think so. If you're 50 and want to go out with a 35-year-old, you can, but decide what you want the relationship to be, and whether that person is going to fulfil your needs. If you wish to travel the world, perhaps somebody at 35 is more focused on their career and they're not going to have the time to do this.

Or maybe you're 50 and with somebody who's 65; perhaps they're secure and set in their ways, and you like being able to do your own thing. Do be honest about your age online. I have friends that worry it's going to scare somebody off, but you don't want the person that's going to be scared off anyway. And you don't want to start out with a lie.

If you've got children, is there ever a right time to introduce a new partner?

You have to make sure there's stability between the two of you before you bring kids into this. So don't rush in too quickly, and wait until the kids are ready too. Don't force it if they're not interested in meeting the person, and keep it casual the first time you introduce them.

Partnership Problems

While we may all dream of living happily ever after, sometimes channels of communication within relationships can break down, and often one party might just stop communicating altogether. This is when resentment can set in, arguments can occur on an almost daily basis, and it can be hard to know if the relationship is worth saving. Many people will have tried couples therapy, others will just have muddled through, but for some a permanent separation or divorce might indeed be the best solution.

RESOLVING CONFLICT

Many people were gobsmacked when, at the tender age of 23, I announced that I was engaged to be married to a man I had met only 11 weeks prior. And yet, over 30 years later, I'm as confident now as I was back then that I made the right decision.

Like most couples, we have often been pushed to the limits: there have been challenges around our own health and that of our family, and pressures of juggling work, finances, running a home, raising children, and coping with ageing parents. Many couples experience additional conflict and strain on their once blooming relationships as they enter midlife, either due to circumstantial reasons, or perhaps because there were always some underlying relationship issues from the get-go; and problems are often masked by the busyness of family life, only bubbling to the surface when there's more time to reflect. But this doesn't necessarily spell the end of the relationship, if we can learn to really listen to each other, make compromises, and find ways to resolve conflict.

And should you come to the realization that your relationship really has reached its conclusion, then it's important to remember that separation or divorce might spell out an end, but it is also a new beginning, and may indeed be the best and most positive path forward.

Couples counselling saved our marriage. My husband and I had a really good marriage throughout our 30s, but as we hit our 40s I began to notice that he had become more depressed, withdrawn, angry, and cold. We spent most of our evenings either arguing or apart, and it got to a point where I was so unhappy that I suggested a temporary separation and counselling.

It was only in therapy that he finally opened up and admitted he'd been keeping a secret that he was too ashamed to tell me about. He had got into serious debt through some bad business advice and wasn't sleeping or talking to anyone about it. I was shocked but told him I loved him and that we could work it through together. Our therapist referred him to the doctor for some CBT, and even recommended a fantastic financial advisor, and over time we have managed to get our marriage back on track.

JANINE, 47

Q & A
Caron Barruw, Psychotherapist specializing
in working with relationships and couples

What can happen with relationships when we reach midlife?

The journey of a relationship is often like that of a sparkler: starting out it's exciting, with the flame shining brightly, but as the years go on, the sparkle starts to dim and that once exciting relationship can start to feel like it has burnt out.

Research backs this up, showing that the initial brain chemistry (high levels of dopamine and norepinephrine, which are released during the early attraction stages) responsible for making us feel giddy, energetic, and often euphoric, reduces over time and after approximately two years it changes significantly.[2]

So what happens after 10 or 20 years?

There are many exceptions, but what usually happens is that a couple tends to follow the well-trodden path of meeting, dating, and then moving in together or getting married. During this time, the focus is mainly on the couple, who enjoy the freedom to grow and develop a life together. But then life gets more complicated, with responsibilities around work and family. Most couples have neither the time or energy to resolve relationship issues at this point, and the demands of everyday life mean that the relationship is left, as I often refer to it, "on the parking lot", unattended to.

By the time we reach midlife and some of this busyness subsides, couples now go back to the parking lot to find their covered, dusty old relationship not looking quite so attractive anymore. And this can often happen right at the same time as menopause comes along for many women. But supporting each other through midlife and menopause can create a stronger couple if both parties are willing and able to navigate the changes together.

Supporting each other through midlife and menopause can create a stronger couple

How do parenting issues contribute to midlife relationship problems?

For those who are able or want to have children, there is a gradual shift in the relationship dynamic: from enjoying being an independent adult couple, focusing all your love and attention on each other, to dividing this between these new little human beings. This responsibility can add huge pressure to a once solid relationship. Cracks may start to appear, often due to an unspoken resentment buried deep inside, around that loss of independence and diversion of our love onto others.

As the parenting years progress, the focus becomes more about the children and their immediate needs, followed swiftly by issues that come with parenting teenagers. As the children leave the nest, many couples start to notice each other again for the first time in a long time. But what was supposed to be a happy period of reunification can often become the biggest crisis of all, as issues that have been hidden or ignored begin to surface.

If our partner is a man, does that affect how we approach conflict resolution?

Without wishing to overgeneralize, a lot of men can feel confused as to what is going on when their relationship starts to break down. And any criticism can feel like a personal attack as they struggle to know how to manage or "fix the problem". They might look for strategies to plaster over the cracks when things go wrong, and need help to learn a different approach, listening to and understanding what their partner is telling them. When it comes to menopause, it is helpful for the couple to educate themselves together as to what they are going through.

How does the menopause impact on relationships?

In the same way that I view marriage, children, and parenting concerns as couple issues, I treat menopause very much as a couple issue. The physical changes are different for every woman, with hot flushes, shifts in mood, issues with libido, and physical problems with intercourse, to name a few, and the relationship between a couple becomes different due to all of these changes.

Many women do not even realize that depression and anxiety are common symptoms of menopause, and weight gain, plummeting self-esteem, and changes in sexual desire hit like a tidal wave. Often the unprepared couple are thrown into a crisis that seems to have no ending.

What can we do to help get our midlife relationships back on track?

No two couples will ever share the same history, and there is no one magic formula to help solve conflict in a relationship. Many couples may struggle to understand what has perhaps gone wrong or changed during the many years since they first met. The key to success is finding a way of expressing to each other how you both feel as you struggle to cope with the changes and challenges that midlife throws your way.

Some couples are not very good at communicating, and both sides can quickly escalate into frustration as various concerns build up unresolved. Teaching couples how to resolve conflict requires both parties to become avid listeners. This enables the "fight or flight" cycle to calm down as both parties will be encouraged to really listen and be heard, and then find a way to compromise.

How can we improve communication?

You need to set up strategies for communication, even though at times the conversations may be incredibly strained and quite often painful too. I use a "toolbox" that includes practical suggestions to help the process to begin. It is not a quick fix; it's a process of rebuilding that enables both partners to grow and develop together.

What happens in a typical couples therapy session?

The goal is to ensure that each person has a space to feel heard. Most couples are in a pattern of communication that does not enable them to resolve conflict. Therapy can identify the triggers in the session and

Conflict Resolution Toolbox

- Take the time in the evenings to be screen-free and to discuss the day's feelings and what has happened, even if only for a few minutes.
- Set date nights to get dressed up and make each other feel special. Make the conversation around both of your needs, and also be sure to have fun.
- Explore sexual options that work for you both to maintain a healthy sex life. Don't be afraid to discuss any issues with your partner, but never dwell on them while actually in bed or during sex.
- Consider couples therapy to resolve the issues that no one talks about.

work with the couple to change reactions, understand each other's point of view – even if they agree to differ, and learn to engage differently.

As the sessions evolve, the therapy unpacks family of origin issues, trauma, bonding, and conflict issues to change patterns within the couple. Therapy usually takes time to achieve the results the couple are looking for, and can often be slower than expected. However, the results are usually long lasting when both people have worked on the relationship.

DIVORCE AND SEPARATION

Sometimes, despite everyone's best efforts, a relationship may be beyond saving and the only option is permanent separation. While this isn't exclusively a midlife issue, it's worth noting that the average age of divorce in most countries is around the mid-40s. I have friends who have got to this point and tell me that even saying the word "divorce" out loud sounds scary, and they have no clue about what they need to do or how they will cope both financially and emotionally on their own.

While ending a relationship can obviously involve a great deal of emotional upheaval, formalizing the termination doesn't have to be such a daunting and terrifying task. If you know the basics, it is much easier to manage, and less stressful to talk about. The practical advice given here relates to divorce law within the UK.

"

Our divorce was ironically the best thing that ever happened to us. We were married very young because I got pregnant at 21 and desperately wanted to keep the baby. We went on to have another child when I was 23, but there was never really any passion in our relationship; we just stayed together for the sake of the kids.

Once both of our kids left home to go to university, although it was scary, we knew we didn't really love each other and agreed to split up. We are still really good friends, and have both been out there dating and travelling the world and doing all the things we missed out on in our 20s. We co-parent really well, and for the first time in such a long time I feel really happy and excited, and am living life to the full.

LUCIA, 46

Q & A
Neil Russell, Head of the Family Department
at Seddons Solicitors

What options are available for couples considering separation?

It's important that you are sure that divorce or separation is really the right way forward for you. There are three options available for all couples:

- You can do nothing; take some time to see if the marriage can be saved.
- If the marriage cannot be saved, then there is the second option of "separation". The terms of a separation can be formalized in a "separation agreement". This is a flexible document that can be tailored to the needs of the couple. It can cover all aspects of the separation including arrangements for the children and the finances. This agreement is not necessarily legally binding but for some couples is a good halfway move until they are ready to proceed with a divorce.
- The third option is divorce. This will provide a couple with finality and lawfully brings the marriage to an end. It is essential to deal with the finances upon divorce. Arrangements for the children can also be dealt with alongside the divorce and finances if necessary.

If any delay in decision-making may risk someone's safety or financial position, we advise that urgent action is taken.

What are the grounds for a divorce?

In the UK, since April 2022, divorce proceedings are now only commenced on the sole ground of "irretrievable breakdown". All that is required is a statement that the marriage has irretrievably broken down. This is referred to as "no-fault divorce".

How long will the process take? And will I have to go to court?

The divorce process itself is paper-based, so no court attendance is necessary. It generally takes between 6–9 months, with most of this time spent waiting for the court to approve the paperwork. Cases can go on for longer, depending on whether the finances and any child arrangements can be agreed between the parties. If not, and court proceedings to address finances are issued, then it can take around 12–18 months to conclusion. You would have to attend court in person if proceedings are issued.

Who should I meet with to arrange a divorce? A mediator or a lawyer?

Generally, it is advisable to meet with a family lawyer before engaging a mediator. They will advise on the process that lies ahead and the options available to you in your specific case. A family lawyer will also be able to recommend mediators who they know to be reliable and effective.

Mediation is not appropriate in all cases, but it can be a useful way to narrow the issues in a cost-effective manner. You can work with your instructed family lawyer alongside the mediation process to ensure that the two can dovetail to achieve a resolution that remains in your best interests.

What will all this cost? Can the state offer any assistance?

There are very limited circumstances in which divorcing parties may qualify for legal aid, but it is always worth checking this with your family lawyer at the outset. Very few family lawyers do legal aid work these days. Your family lawyer should provide you with detailed costs estimates at the start of your case, and give you regular updates so that you know the cost to you at all stages.

The likely cost is dependent on the issues to be resolved; for example, whether an early financial settlement can be reached and/or whether there are additional aspects to be resolved, such as child arrangements. There are some "divorce loans" available to meet legal fees, and their suitability can be discussed depending on your circumstances. Sometimes it is possible to get your partner to fund your costs. The key thing is that there should be a level playing field, where possible.

What am I entitled to with regard to financial settlement?

There's no simple answer as to what you are entitled to upon divorce. This will need to take into account the resources you and your spouse have between you, the individual needs of you and your spouse, as well as any children of the marriage. The decision will be based upon the individual facts of your case, and your family lawyer will be able to advise you upon what you may be entitled to.

It may be that interim financial support is needed by one party from the other while the divorce process is going through. Again, your family lawyer can advise if this is relevant for you, and if so, how to secure this support.

What are the usual arrangements regarding children?

The welfare of any children of the family is the priority in all divorce/separation cases. Where possible, you will be encouraged to reach an agreement with your spouse about children. This is the

The Divorce Process

There are a number of steps in the divorce process in the UK, and your role will depend on whether you are filing for divorce or whether your partner is filing for divorce.

STEP 1: FILING FOR DIVORCE

Sole application

One party will need to file a Divorce Application, which is generally done online. The person who files the application then becomes the "Applicant" in the divorce proceedings. There is a court fee for filing the divorce application.

- The other party will be served with the court issued divorce application and a blank Acknowledgement of Service form. This party then becomes the "Respondent" to the divorce proceedings.
- The Respondent must complete the online Acknowledgement of Service form and send this back to the court within 14 days.
- Once the Respondent has replied to the court with their completed Acknowledgement of Service, the divorce application will be issued by the court.

Joint application

Both parties can decide to submit a Joint Divorce Application. In this case, the procedure is the same as if it were a sole application, with the only difference being that one of the parties is referred to as "Applicant 1" and the other party is referred to as "Applicant 2".

STEP 2: CONDITIONAL ORDER

- After the issue of the application for divorce you must wait 20 weeks before you can apply for the first of the two-part divorce order, called the Conditional Order. In the application for the Conditional Order, you must confirm that everything in the divorce application remains unchanged and you wish to proceed with the divorce.
- Once the Applicant has applied for the Conditional Order, the court will set a date for the pronouncement of Conditional Order. This is the interim stage of divorce. The divorce isn't finalized yet, but this stage is important for arranging financial matters.

STEP 3: FINAL ORDER

- The Applicant is entitled to apply for Final Order six weeks and one day after the date of Conditional Order. If the Applicant does not apply, the Respondent can apply 12 weeks after the date by which the Applicant could have applied.
- Once six weeks and one day have elapsed from the day the Conditional Order was pronounced (not less than 26 weeks and one day from the date of the divorce application), you will be able to apply for the final divorce order. It is not until the Final Order is made that your marriage is ended, and only then are you formally divorced. NB: you should always take specialist legal advice before applying for Final Order.

most cost-effective approach and allows for greater flexibility. Generally, it also means a more amicable resolution, which is in the best interests of the child(ren).

Mediation can be helpful in reaching agreements for the children, and in some cases, family therapy is advised. If an agreement cannot be reached, then an application to the court can be made for a Child Arrangements Order and/or Specific Issue Order. This will formally determine the arrangements for the children. However, the starting point in relation to the children is for the parties to first try to reach an agreement.

Who gets the house in a divorce?

The family home has a special place within the finances. The decision about the family home will consider a number of factors. These will include the housing needs of the children, the housing needs of you and your spouse, and whether there are other assets and resources available to one or both parties. Again, all of this will be specific to each case so your family lawyer will be able to explain what this might mean for you.

If I don't currently work, will I be compelled to find a job?

Non-working spouses may be encouraged to return to work in certain cases. However, it is not always possible for this to happen immediately, or sometimes at all. This will depend on the circumstances, but the court will look at earning capacity, not just income.

What if my partner leaves the country?

If one party leaves the country they can still be served with court proceedings but rules for service may be different. If a party leaves with a view to hiding assets, you can apply to the court for a Freezing Order. This will preserve the assets so they remain properly available for sharing in any financial remedy proceedings.

Do you have any final words of advice?

Going through a divorce can be one of the most stressful and anxious times in a person's life, so it is important that your case is dealt with carefully and in a way that will best help you to move on as smoothly as possible.

You might want to work with a therapist to support you with the breakdown of your marriage, and your lawyer or doctor may be able to recommend a suitable therapist. Remember, divorce shouldn't be about taking revenge, it should be about moving forward.

However painful a divorce may be, a new beginning could be the best thing to happen to you. It's not uncommon for a marriage to break down over a period of time, and each person may go on to do so much better when separated than they did in the marriage.

Friendships

If I've learnt one thing over the past half century it is that there are friends, there is family, and then there are friends that become family. The best friends know you inside and out, warts and all, and will forever support you, lift you up, and will always have your back, no matter what. Of course, there are also friends who may fall by the wayside, for all sorts of reasons, and at times losing touch can be painful, complicated, and confusing, yet this is an area in our lives that nobody really talks about. This chapter gives focus to the importance of friendships, and how to navigate their inevitable ups and downs.

NAVIGATING FRIENDSHIPS IN MIDLIFE

Life can get busy and complicated, and quite often it can be difficult to find the time to nurture and maintain our friendships. And how do you go about making new friends if perhaps you have had to relocate, have never been fortunate enough to find a strong friendship circle, or maybe have grown apart and don't get on with them anymore?

With so many demands on us midlifers, it's natural to prioritize who gets and needs our attention first, and for those of you with partners, children, ageing parents, and demanding colleagues, being a good friend can often end up feeling like yet another responsibility.

Some friends will be understanding, perhaps in the same boat as you, whereas others may be more needy and less forgiving if they hardly ever see or hear from you. So how can we still enjoy each other's company, and ensure we show up for each other as and when we need to?

I sadly lost my husband last year and if it wasn't for my amazing girlfriends all rallying around to help me through that time, I don't know what I would have done. I don't have any siblings, so my friends are literally like my sisters, we do everything together and they include me in all of their family celebrations too. They have helped me to process my grief and have given me the strength and courage to look forward and plan for a future I hadn't quite expected.

SANDRA, 59

Q & A
Claire Cohen, Award-winning Journalist and Author

Why are female friendships so important in midlife?

Female friendships can sustain women in ways that even romantic relationships cannot, and studies at the University of Oxford have found that women get more emotional intimacy and have more in common with their female friends.[3]

Midlife can be a golden time for female friendship. By now, the myth that we should all have one perfect "best friend forever" has probably started to fade, and even if you do have one very close friend, you'll probably also have gathered a group of other women from different areas of life. That support system, however small or big, can really start to come into its own.

Within your friendships over the years there may have been toxic dynamics, friendships that ended, and those who drifted away, and you'll now have a clearer idea of the sort of friends who are right for you. You'll also have dealt with a lot of life and learnt to lean on other people, to be vulnerable and ask for support. This openness is a key building block of friendship and much harder to achieve when you're younger, but it's what elevates your female friendships into relationships that are critical to your survival: they're the people you go to when making life's big decisions.

Can longstanding friendships survive the tests of time?

Old friends from our younger years and friendships forged in the fire of first jobs or parenthood are some of the most precious bonds in our lives, and shared history is a powerful thing. But they can also be some of the most frustrating, at times. The friends you made while growing up knew you when you were an unfinished version of the person you are today. The friends you made when you started work or had your first child got to know you at a time of upheaval and growth.

The oxygen of many such friendships is space: giving each other room to keep growing, accepting that the other person won't stay the same forever.

Why do some manage to hold on to lifelong friendships and others find it hard to hold on to many at all?

You never really know how many friends someone else has. Social media in particular has allowed us to create worlds of illusion, where someone might appear to be surrounded by friends, but how do you know they have a good enough friend to pick up the phone to during hard times? But I know how turbulent female friendship can be, and how it can feel as though no one wants to remain friends with you while other people have lifelong best friends.

Looking back over friendships that I thought would last forever but didn't, a common factor was that it had all been quite superficial. I had thought the "real" me was someone that other people might not like, so I had been the friend I thought they wanted. Of course, this meant that I wasn't being authentic, vulnerable, and open – all the things that are the cement of long-lasting friendship.

Do friendships naturally start to drop off in midlife?

I think that as we hurtle towards midlife, friendships can fall down our list of priorities as we put our partners, family, and work first. But that's not your fault: society has undervalued female friendship for centuries and sold us the romantic fairy tale instead of the platonic one.

Can you have *too many* friends in your life?

As we get older, the quality becomes more important than quantity. That said, keeping channels for new or deeper friendship open is a healthy way to live. According to research done by Professor Robin Dunbar, a friendship expert and evolutionary anthropologist at the University of Oxford, the maximum number of "social contacts" any person can cope with is 150.[4]

This may sound like a lot, but when you count family, close friends, casual friends, colleagues, acquaintances, friends of friends you see sometimes, it all adds up. We group these people into friendship "circles", and people can move towards the middle (where our closest friends sit) or towards the edges at different times. Extroverts may relish the entire group and spread themselves thinly, while introverts might concentrate on a small, closer set. You'll find your own balance.

How can we bring up difficult issues of friends upsetting us?

We'd all prefer to avoid having awkward conversations with friends, and worry that rocking the boat might cause irreparable damage. But the worst thing we can do in a friendship is to not address something, letting resentment simmer and build.

So have the conversation, and plan what you're going to say. It's a good idea to set expectations, beginning with something like, "This is really hard to say to you, but it's important because our friendship means so much to me." Or "I wasn't sure how to bring this up because I didn't want to hurt you, but I want us to have a totally honest friendship." You can't predict or control how your friend will react, you just have to listen and be prepared for them to act defensively. But if you're respectful and let them know you're doing this because you want to find a solution, you hopefully will.

It's never too late to make new friends. I've interviewed women in their 90s who are still forging new friendships.

—

How can we recognize when a friendship becomes toxic or unhelpful?

It's really not always easy to spot when a friendship has turned toxic. To me, a toxic friendship is one in which there is a permanent imbalance of power: the other person always demands to have things their way, to do what they want to do. They make you feel small. They judge you. You don't feel able to confide in them or have to hide parts of yourself in case they get upset or angry. They might resent your good news or be jealous.

But it might not be that extreme: you might just have a friend who pushes you to have a drink when you'd rather not; who loves to gossip about mutual pals; or who tries to buy your affection. It's that drip, drip, drip of negative interactions that make you feel drained or exhausted when you see them. If that happens more often than not, it's worth examining the dynamic of that friendship and asking whether it's right for you.

How do we move away from these friendships without hurting feelings?

Not all friendships last forever: some are destined to only have a cameo role in your life, and that's fine. The difficulty arises when the desire to end a friendship isn't mutual. It might seem that the "easiest" path is simply to ghost or cut off a friend, even one you've known for decades, ending the friendship quickly and without a major drama. We often convince ourselves that this is the kindest way to go about it, but that's a lie: this is really hurtful. We have to tell the truth and explain to the friend why the friendship no longer works.

How easy is it to make new friends post 40?

It's never too late to make new friends. I've interviewed women in their 90s who are still forging new friendships. It's often at life's pinch points that we might seek new friendships: after a divorce, house move, or bereavement. Sometimes, you find you're temporarily not on the same page as your friends, if they are busy dealing with family or a new job, and you might feel lonely and look for someone new to spend time with.

I do think you need to be deliberate about making new friends. This means putting yourself out there. One woman I know posted in an online group set up specifically for women in her city to make new connections, which helped her make one good friend and several acquaintances she can call on. Another booked a trip with a women-only travel group, telling herself that, at worst, she'd have a great holiday and meet some new people, but ended up making two new friends that she now regularly travels with. Too many of us just expect friendships to happen organically, when the truth is that you have to put the effort in.

Family Matters

For those of us who are part of the "sandwich generation", juggling care for both our parents and children can bring enormous pressures. When we reach this stage of our lives, our children are likely to be tweenagers or young adults, and caring for their emotional needs can be even more challenging when both we and they were younger. Perhaps our own ageing parents might be struggling with a range of concerning health conditions, and there are worries about how to support them when they are left on their own, maybe after suffering a bereavement. It can sometimes feel like we never stop worrying.

PARENTING IN MIDLIFE

I could write an entire book from personal experience on what to expect with a house full of tweens/teenagers/young adults: from issues around bullying, trolling, vaping, smoking, and drinking to relationship breakups, health concerns, dropping out of university, starting job searching, and young married life. I've been there, and bought all the T-shirts.

It's important to acknowledge that the times are very different to when we were younger, and growing up in a digital world, continually bombarded with images of the "perfect" lives of others on social media, takes its toll on our children. We are also a generation of "helicopter parents" who have perhaps coddled our kids, with "positive parenting" star charts and a "well done for breathing" style of parenting. Is it really any wonder that they are perhaps now finding navigating through life more challenging than we did?

When you are supporting a child who is struggling with their mental (or physical) health, no matter how old they are, it is natural to almost absorb their symptoms as your own. We feel their pain, and at times it can be all consuming. As a mum of four, I can attest that I rarely get to feel truly worry-free. But it's vitally important to try to find ways to stop blurring the lines between what they are feeling and experiencing and what *you* are feeling and experiencing.

Your role is to be the adult, the person who can lend an ear whenever they need you, and direct them to professional help if it's required. But if you get to a point where you find yourself lying awake at night constantly worrying, feeling anxious and even scared about their future, you are likely to become unwell yourself, and that's not going to be helpful to them at all.

So try to find ways to offload and look after your own mental health, whether that's through walking and talking with friends or your partner, joining support groups online or in person, or even going on a mental health first aid course, where you will learn how to help someone you care about while putting boundaries in place to protect yourself.

Q & A
Leanne Cowan, Chartered Clinical
Psychologist and Founder of KindleKids

Why can midlife parenting be more challenging than in our younger years?

During midlife we are going through a range of hormonal changes that affect our mood, sense of competence, and capacity to cope. Menopause also often coincides with parenting tweens or teenagers and perhaps caring for ageing relatives too. At the same time that we may be battling anxiety, sleep deprivation, and loss of self-esteem, our children are often experiencing hormonal surges, mood swings, and questions about their own identity.

Children's developmental goal is to separate from their parents and forge their own path. This in turn affects their mood, engagement, and capacity to cope. Teenagers will often require enhanced, sensitive parental support just at the point when our maternal resources are reduced. These conflicting needs can create a perfect storm, albeit usually temporary, within the family dynamic.

Are "challenging" behaviours just a normal part of adolescence?

Learning how to recognize, understand, and manage different emotions allows a child to develop their confidence and resilience. Thinking back to your own teenage years, you may recall a sense that you knew more about how the world worked and a belief that your parents did not "get you". You may have rallied against parental boundaries and wished that they could just be less "controlling" and "embarrassing". As hard as it can be to accept, this may be what your own teenage children feel about you now. There is no need to take this personally as it is a normal developmental process.

You also have to consider the added influence of social media, misinformation, and exposure to many, often conflicting values. It is therefore no surprise that this can be one of the most tumultuous parenting stages. However, rest assured that over time most parents go on to have healthy, happy, and connected relationships with their older teens and adult children.

What should we do when our children don't want our help?

As mothers, we generally wish for our children to live happy, successful, and autonomous lives. When they seem to be struggling, we can feel upset, powerless, and overwhelmed. If we are experiencing menopause simultaneously, we may struggle to problem solve, and it can be difficult to know how, when, or even if we should help.

While needing support, teenagers may complain that they are being micro-managed, and not shown sufficient trust. They may become oppositional and reject any efforts to guide or assist them. The phrase I hear most often from parents is that "they don't know how to help", and parents may be left feeling de-skilled in supporting their children. This can be complicated further when children have moved out or gone away to university and are expected to manage their own finances and routine for perhaps the first time. Even if they are feeling overwhelmed, they may not want to admit this to their parents.

When children are struggling, they will often direct their anger and upset towards you. Parents will be castigated, often for events that they have no direct responsibility for. Even when parents provide appropriate support and advice, they must run the gauntlet of rejection first. These responses, as distressing as they are, reflect a normal developmental process. Our offspring will feel compelled to be autonomous and "live their best life" while also needing parental validation, reassurance, and acceptance. This requires a leap of faith. When children are their most demanding and menopausal mothers are low in resources, we, as parents, still need to provide unconditional love and support.

How can we help our children navigate mental health challenges?

Most teenagers will experience periods of anxiety, self-doubt, and depressed thinking as they navigate adolescence. However, this does not necessarily indicate a serious issue or a need for formal psychological therapy.

These challenges are a natural part of growing up as our children work out who they are and the kind of adult that they want to become. However, if you are worried about your child, there are practical things that you can do to support them.

To help your child, they will need to feel connected to you and to be able to communicate openly with you. However, parents may struggle to maintain open and effective communication with their teenagers, who may be less inclined to share their thoughts and feelings.

If your children do not talk to you about what's going on in their lives, this does not make you a bad parent, it may just mean they are less comfortable with expressing difficult feelings. In this situation, letting them know that you are there to support them and will do whatever it takes to help can be enough. Being a nonjudgemental and steady presence can provide enough stability for some children to navigate their teenage years; they will already feel more contained, resilient, and able to cope with life's challenges.

When children are their most demanding and menopausal mothers are low in resources, we, as parents, still need to provide unconditional love and support.

—

When might it be time to hand over to a professional?

Many challenges of adolescence are an expected part of growing up, and obviously not all bouts of anger, anxiety, and poor choices need intervention from a professional. When concerned about their child, many parents take the "wait and see" approach. While this works for lots of children, especially if their distress is situational, such as due to a friendship issue or subject that they are having trouble learning, it is also important to be mindful of when more intervention may be needed.

There are a number of indicators to look out for when deciding whether professional support is needed. If your child is consistently avoiding activities that used to bring them pleasure or has changed from being an outgoing teen to one that cannot eat, sleep, wash, or get out of bed, it would be time to seek external advice. Self-harm, disordered eating, extreme recreational drug use, or expressing a wish to die are all red flags that require immediate attention.

How can we get a diagnosis and referral to access the right help?

Though there are several different ways to access support, finding the right professional can be a minefield. While there are many very good and ethical professionals, it's important to note that just because someone calls themselves a psychologist it doesn't mean they are. There are many people working with teenagers, young adults, and even children who claim to be psychologists and therapists but have very little training or experience.

If you should choose to take your child to a psychotherapist, psychologist, coach, or counsellor, ensure they are registered with the most appropriate professional regulating body, which for psychologists in the UK is the HCPC (Health and Care Professions Council), and for other types of therapists, such as psychotherapists or counsellors, may be the UKCP (United Kingdom Council for Psychotherapy) or BACP (British Association for Counselling and Psychotherapy).

If you are concerned, usually the first place to go is your doctor as they can refer you to appropriate services. Unfortunately, waiting times can be very long and this can be frustrating as we want to support our children and get them what they need as soon as possible. When families can afford it or have medical insurance, they may choose to find an independent psychologist.

A clinical psychologist is a good place to start as they will assess your child's emotional wellbeing and any support that they may need, and can direct you to the best place to get this. Young Minds has an array of helpful resources and advice, as does our KindleKids website (see p.249).

CARING FOR AGEING PARENTS

Many women tell me that caring for their ageing and often unwell parents can be a full-time and incredibly demanding job. Some women have had to leave their own jobs, and find themselves neglecting their partners and children to focus on the needs of their parents. This is especially true for those who cannot afford private care, or are having to prop up the care service that is being provided by their local authorities.

According to Carers UK, informal care saves the UK around £162 billion per year,[5] and the number of unpaid carers is 5.7 million.[6] The entire care system in this country relies on us midlifers providing that extra support, and without us the system would collapse. But the impact of juggling these demands can seriously affect our own wellbeing, so it's really important to factor in time for self-care and garner support from others so that these demands don't swallow you up and leave you feeling frazzled and unable to cope.

Support groups that meet in person or online, like The Latte Lounge, are really good places to connect with others who may be going through something similar. Being able to swap advice or just share worries can be extremely helpful, a place for you to unburden yourself.

But there can come a point where you might no longer be the best person to provide care, and navigating the options can be overwhelming. A common concern is how to ensure our parents' interests are taken care of should they become incapacitated, allowing us to advocate for them and make decisions on their behalf (such as getting a Lasting Power of Attorney, or LPA). Understanding the various courses of action and what help is available can make this difficult time less stressful.

My father was diagnosed with a degenerative illness last year, and unfortunately my mum was not of capacity to make vital and measured decisions as she has dementia, so my siblings and I were advised to arrange a health and wealth LPA for my father while he still could make decisions. I'm so pleased we did, as it was quite a lengthy process, and it means that now he can't get out of the house to the bank or the doctor easily we are able to advocate for him and for my mum about their finances and medical records.

LYNNE, 59

Q & A
Jackie Gray, Founder of The Carents Room

What are "Carents"?

Those who find themselves as the primary carers for their elderly parents. Despite playing such a vital role, it is recognized that carents are largely unsupported by the state and find it difficult to access good information, advice, products, and services that could make life easier for them and their parents. This is what led me to set up The Carents Room.

Combining family care and paid work can lead to increased stress, family conflict, and financial pressures. Many of these factors can have negative implications on the caregiver's health, wellbeing, and often their ability to remain in work. Many carers therefore reduce their hours, which can have significant consequences for their own finances and retirement prospects.

Why are these substantial caring responsibilities often falling to midlife women?

With funding for adult social care not keeping pace with the growing numbers of older people needing care, numbers of care home beds are actually falling, and government policy in the UK has promoted supporting people in their own homes. What this means is that lots of midlife women are increasingly shouldering much of the burden of caring for elderly parents, often at a time when many women:

- still have parental responsibilities of their own
- are developing their own health problems and experiencing menopause
- are at the peak of their career and working towards pensions and retirement
- have new responsibilities for grandchildren
- might be coping with changes in status due to divorce or bereavement

Care Support Available

- **Health services:** from hospital-based specialist doctors, nurses, and therapists through to multidisciplinary community teams and everyday support from the primary healthcare team based at a doctor's surgery.
- **Assessment:** to help establish financial and care needs and assistance.
- **Adapting the home:** help with installing ramps, grab rails, shower seats, commodes, and so on.
- **Monitors** and monitoring services.
- **Personal care services:** help with everyday tasks such as dressing, eating, and taking medicine.

What is the first step toward accessing support?

In the UK, you can access support from your Local Authority by contacting the Adult Social Care team directly, or ask your doctor to make a referral on your behalf. Local authorities are legally required to provide the following.

- A needs assessment to determine what help your parents actually need. However, they will only get that help if they meet stringent financial thresholds.
- A financial assessment to ascertain whether your parents meet the criteria to qualify for different aspects of care.
- A carers' assessment examines your needs as a carer and is means tested.

How can I get help to adapt the home if needed?

Depending on where you live, these services are variably provided by local authority adults social care services and NHS Community Rehabilitation teams. A call to your council will direct you to the right place and you are likely to get a good and quick response. A home visit, to understand what your parents need, will be followed by free installation and supply of all the necessary equipment. This service is NOT means tested; items are loaned free of charge within a limited budget. In many areas, expensive items such as stairlifts will not be included.

EXPERT ADVICE
JANE BUTLER, EDITORIAL INFORMATION MANAGER, CARERS UK

Caring for ageing parents can be challenging as their needs become more complex. However, there are various ways you can support your parents to be as independent as possible. You can find more guidance and practical advice on each of these on the Carers UK website (see p.249).

1. **Talk to your parents** If they need extra help to keep on top of everyday tasks, you could suggest small changes at first to lighten their load. The role reversal that involves you taking care of your parents might take some time to adjust to on both sides, so taking small steps is a good approach. Discussing options with your parents, if possible, and providing choices about what changes could be made will help to make them feel more comfortable and involved with decisions.

2. **Adapt the home environment** As we get older, there's a higher risk of falling and developing issues with our balance. It's important to look out for tripping hazards within the home, from rugs to slippy floor surfaces. There are many ways the home can be adapted to help prevent falls, from installing grab rails to non-slip mats. Arranging a review to see whether any adjustments are needed, with the assistance of an occupational therapist, could be helpful.

3. **Consider professional support** You may have reached a point where the support you or other family members can give isn't enough – many carers find they reach a stage of burnout and exhaustion. Having professionals to help is a way of taking some pressure off your own shoulders so you can look after your health and support them in other ways. Looking at professional care can be a difficult shift to come to terms with, but it should be one that benefits everybody involved.

4. **Think ahead** Nobody wants to think about a time when they won't be able to make their own choices in the future, but putting plans in place as early as possible can save much stress further down the line. There are several different options to explore, from making a power of attorney to arranging an advance statement (which allows you to record the care you would like in the future).

Can the local authority also provide monitors and monitoring equipment?

As part of the service relating to adapting the home, most areas will also provide home monitoring equipment, which will ensure that your parents can get rapid help in the face of problems such as becoming ill, collapsing, or falling. Depending on your parents' financial circumstances, this equipment and the related support might be provided free of charge, but it is likely to be means tested and may incur a monthly fee.

You can also install your own monitoring equipment, but you and your parents will need to be clear about who will be contacted and what will happen should they become unwell.

What are the various care services that are available?

The level of care people need varies dramatically: some might only need occasional support with food shopping, whereas others might be bed-bound and need around the clock supervision and help to eat and stay clean. There are different types of care services, and the main ones include:

- **Home care services:** these provide short visits to people's homes to help with food preparation, dressing, and bathing (but don't include all the assistance that might be required, such as shopping).
- **Live-in care services:** carers live in a person's home, providing 24/7 care – these are less common.
- **Residential care services**: these are care homes and nursing homes.

Care is expensive, and it doesn't take long to eat into lifetime savings. Live-in care services can be slightly cheaper than residential care homes but rely on suitable accommodation. Home visits are a cheaper option still, but, generally, home care services don't help with everything; you will usually have to source support for things like house cleaning, maintenance, gardening, utilities, and possibly shopping separately.

All care services are registered with a national regulator (see p.249). The regulators will provide a directory of registered suppliers in your location along with the results of their inspection reports.

How can we decide on which care service is right for us?

If your parents qualify for financial assistance then you will be able to discuss and work with their social worker to ensure that the services provided by the local authority meet their needs and preferences. If your parents cannot get financial assistance then you will need to find and organize an appropriate care service for them. Whatever type of care you're considering, keep in mind the points detailed opposite.

ALL CARE SERVICES

- Use the relevant inspection directory to find services in the area.
- Get "word of mouth" feedback.
- Be wary of published client feedback: negative comments won't be included.
- Check the regulator's inspection report: few services are "excellent", but many are "good"; think carefully about services that "need improvement".
- Be prepared to shop around.

HOME CARE

- Ask about additional prices for cover at weekends and bank holidays.
- Attend a "home-based assessment" appointment so that you can help your parent explain their needs and understand what your role will be.
- Consider how care staff will be able to access your parents' home, and any security and insurance arrangements.
- Discuss how the service will ensure that the same care workers visit, to enable familiarity and avoid a trail of strangers entering the home.
- Check how they will get in touch to tell you about any changes to the care arrangements (timing, people, price).
- Ask what contingency arrangements will be put in place in case a care worker is late or misses a visit.
- Request assurance that the care workers have had the right training.
- Find out how you can adjust the care package or provide feedback.

RESIDENTIAL CARE

- Don't judge at face value: beautiful bedding and whitewashed walls do not guarantee loving care.
- Ask about staff: high turnover is an indicator of a problem provider and will not be pleasant for your parents.
- Ask about any "hidden" costs and how price hikes will be managed for the duration.
- Remember, once a poorly parent in need of care is a resident, it is very hard to move them elsewhere.
- Be prepared to compromise.
- Consider location carefully: while a parent might want to stay local, you need to consider your visits, and long commutes can be stressful.
- Visit the home at random and unscheduled times to get a real sense of the service rather than the intentionally presented version.
- Safeguarding can be an issue in any institutional setting. Keep checking with your parents, "Do you feel safe?"
- Think about the future: homes provide different levels of care, and if your parents are likely to need nursing care or dementia care, find out if this will be available onsite or if a major transfer elsewhere will be necessary.
- Consider local doctor's services: it is likely that your parents will need these, and some are better than others.

Grief

The loss of someone close to you, no matter the circumstances or their age, propels you into a totally new and frightening place where love is replaced by loss, and the world we once knew and felt safe in suddenly feels strange and frightening. I doubt there will be many of you reading this that haven't at some point experienced the loss of a loved one. And as we reach our 40s, 50s, and beyond, there will no doubt be concerns around ageing parents and perhaps even our own partners, and how we will feel or cope if we were to lose them.

DEALING WITH LOSS

At the time of writing this, I'm blessed to have both my parents alive, but I have sadly lost good friends along the way. Because I wasn't offered any support to deal with the experience at the time, I created unhealthy coping mechanisms. Grief leads you to a place where you are forced to consider the meaning of life. But whatever type of loss you may have suffered, there really is no right or wrong way or appropriate time frame in which to grieve.

Many women struggle to know how, where, or when to get help with loss, and wonder if they'll ever go back to feeling "normal" again. For some it could take weeks or months, for others it could take years, or perhaps they never "get over" it. It's important to get the help and support you need as soon as you need it, rather than letting it go unchecked, as I did for years.

This chapter will help you to understand the different stages and types of grief, discover how to access help so that you can find healthy ways to cope (or help others to cope), and learn to adjust to your new reality and perhaps even emerge stronger from the experience.

Peter and I had met and married within a year at the age of 25. He was my rock, my best friend, and my soul mate. We did everything together and were pretty inseparable throughout our life. He was the most amazing father to our three kids, and always there for any of us or anyone who needed him.

Five years ago, out of the blue, he was diagnosed with leukaemia and passed away within six months. My world was torn apart. I couldn't function at all for the first year, but thanks to my incredible children and close friends supporting me and encouraging me to get some bereavement support, I slowly managed to find a way to adjust to life without him.

Life will obviously never be the same as it was, but I have managed to find many moments of light within the dark. I have learnt to play bridge for the first time in my life, I have been on some amazing girls' holidays abroad, I have started volunteering for a grief charity, and I am also a new grandma, pouring my love into this new little life. I think my husband would be very proud of the way I have somehow managed to cope without him.

TESSA, 55

Q & A
Dr Shelley Gilbert MBE, Psychotherapist and
Founder of Grief Encounter, a bereavement support charity

How do most of us experience grief?

Grief is a natural response to losing someone we love. But we need to reframe the way we think about it. We often meet the misguided and outdated notion of many "stages of bereavement", and the idea that we have to pass through these in a set order to finally reach acceptance and "let go" of a loved one.

However, grief is non-linear, and it is better to replace the idea of stages with a picture of an "upward spiral" of grief. This model allows bereaved people to accept and face their feelings, knowing that these will continue to come and go, but with less intensity over time.

What is the "upward spiral" of grief?

The spiral includes the commonly known feelings of grief: disbelief, denial, shock, sadness, guilt, despair, and anger, but does not set them in any particular order. Looking at grief in this way allows for the ebb and flow of these emotions and:

- takes away the pressure of the "stages", making it less frightening for people to revisit the feelings time and time again
- gives the bereaved permission to grieve in their own way, over time

How do we begin to work through grief?

It is important to first understand the difference between the two phases of grief. Although we call them phase 1 and 2, they're not mutually exclusive. Phase 1 addresses the initial trauma and traumatic response to it (in other words the "fight, flight, freeze, fragment" model). That's when we are propelled into survival mode, where it can feel like you are in a black hole, trapped even.

Phase 2 is where we don't need to be in that traumatic response phase anymore, but can allow access to more cognitive thinking. This is when you are not constantly feeling in danger, but there's still a presence of something lurking. Then, you can process the grief. Grief lasts forever: the raw, acute pain doesn't.

How long can we expect to grieve for?

It takes time to adjust to the new realities you face. It's important to highlight that this process is not so much about letting go, but adjustment, remembrance, and constructively filling the void. Grieving is a complex process, full of confusions and pitfalls that can easily lead to destructive patterns and depleted resilience.

The Upward Spiral of Grief

The spiral model highlights the difference between the traumatic impact of death (Phase 1) and the longer-term work of learning to live without the person who has died (Phase 2).

- **Phase 1:** this initial "traumatic" response can feel like you're in a black hole. The tough part is finding your way out when all seems so dark.
- **Phase 2:** you'll be moving round, knowing that there will be more, grey, white, and black days ahead, even some that will allow the colour back in. As you work through your grief, you'll find that you can control some of your feelings and thoughts. And they'll be less intense. Warning signs include being stuck, or operating at extremes.

When should we worry about our feelings, thoughts, and behaviours?

We share similar feelings following a bereavement, however not necessarily at the same time or in the same way as others. The bereaved and those close to them need to look out for and be concerned about feelings such as being stuck in a state of abject fear – the initial terror that you experience following your traumatic grief as you're propelled into an unsafe world. That's a very lonely place,

and one of deep isolation. Many of us may feel guilt that our loved one has gone and we are still here, and that needs to be unpacked in a safe way, at the right time. Sometimes, we are afraid to bring our feelings up. Or perhaps we don't have the right words to explain the depths of despair or even joyful feelings. Perhaps we feel abandoned, too alone, and unsafe.

How can we offer support to the bereaved, or find support ourselves?

Some people can take a long time to ask for help, and there are deep reasons, conscious and unconscious, for that. But there is no right or wrong timeline when it comes to asking for and getting help. Some people may never seek help, and try to work through their grief in private; others may struggle so much that they feel that reaching out for help is essential.

We need to find ways to open up the conversations around help and support, rather than trying to shut them down for fear of making things worse. There are many simple ways of showing support to others after a bereavement, usually by assessing their immediate needs and response to the traumatic impact. In most cases, it's about offering them food, shelter, love, and warmth at first. If you have suffered a bereavement, you don't usually need to ask friends and family for help, they will probably offer it in spades to begin with; but at some point, maybe when the reality has kicked in and you're

Memory-making is helpful and important: cherishing memories from the past, the present, and into the future.

—

feeling especially low, but people have stopped coming around all the time, that's when you can dip quite far. This is when asking your doctor for recommendations of counselling or self-care can be helpful, or get in touch with grief specialists like Grief Encounter (see p.249).

What practical things can we do to help ourselves?

There are both public and private ways in which people can help themselves: journalling, telling your story in creative ways; reading and writing poetry; being more physical and grounded, with nature activities; and trying new and different challenges and groups. Always remember that support can come from surprising sources if you reach out.

Do we ever really accept the loss?

The word "acceptance" is tricky: if we are really honest, it's so hard to accept the forever loss, but we can learn to live with it and change our life accordingly. It's about how we can move forward to transform the pain and grief. And there are lots of ways to do that with the right support network. Some people prefer to do that privately with a counsellor, whereas others may prefer to do it in a more public space with others who have been through something similar.

Dealing with the reality of death is very foreign, so we need to think about those

Recovering From Loss

DO

- Be alert for warning signs about being stuck in the traumatic response stage.
- Be kind to yourself.
- Treasure past memories, but also focus on the present and future.
- Stay connected, both with yourself and with others.
- Remember that grieving is complex, confusing, and hard work.
- Find a range of trusted resources for self-help and from others.
- Hold the hope that things will be better.
- Remind yourself that the world is ever-changing, but human nature doesn't.

DON'T

- Suffer in silence, you do not have to manage everything alone.
- Lose your sense of humour and ability to have fun at times.
- Pour out your grief on social media; use it wisely.
- Think time is the only measure of grief.

existential questions about the meaning of life and how we are going to live the rest of our lives in a different way, and not be scared of that. In moving forward, I find that memory-making is helpful and important: cherishing memories from the past, the present, and into the future.

WORK & FINANCES

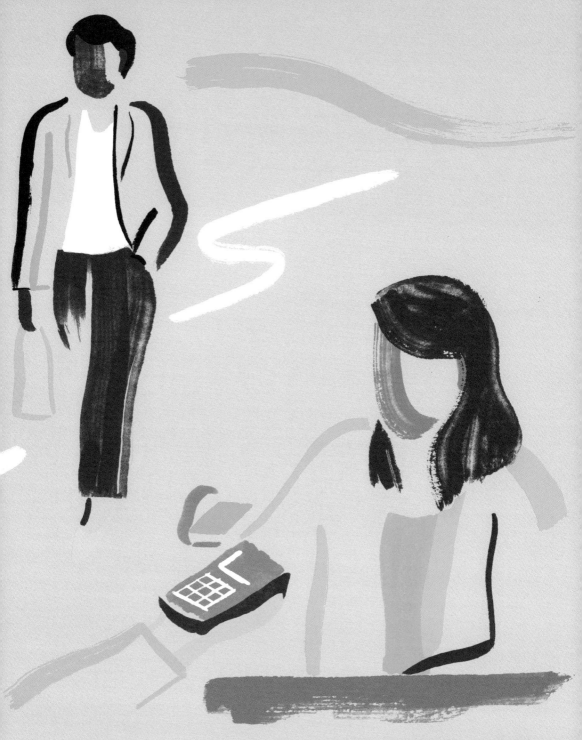

216 — 241

Work Life

Midlife is the perfect time to reflect on where we are professionally: our goals are unlikely to be the same as when we started out in our careers. But women can often find that they are struggling to achieve an elusive work–life balance, or that they no longer enjoy the work they are doing but don't know how to make a change. Sometimes they might find it hard to get back into working after a career break. Now is the time to press pause and do a "stock take", to consider what's working and what's not.

ASSESSING YOUR CAREER IN MIDLIFE

Perhaps you've worked your way to the top of the ladder and are not sure where to go next. Maybe you are happy to continue working at the level you are at, but in a totally different company or industry. Are you returning to work after a break, or looking for a new challenge? You might have gotten to a stage where you have more financial security and want to cut back on work or take time out to do something that would give you more fulfilment, rather than just working to pay the bills.

Throughout your life you may, at some point, have thought about a career change. It wouldn't be surprising. After all, in most countries you have to make decisions on what you're going to do for the rest of your life when you're 16. However, as we get older and become more confident and more established in our careers, we know more about what we love doing and what we don't, and our life circumstances will have likely changed dramatically. It's not unusual to find ourselves entering midlife feeling less than enamoured with our "chosen" career path.

I certainly know that teenage Katie is very different to midlife Katie, and what I love, am good at, and need right now is nothing like when I started out. And for those of you who perhaps stayed at home to bring up a young family for a number of years or who have been made redundant, there may be a gap in employment on your résumé, making a return to work feel daunting. But this can also be an incredibly exciting and liberating time.

I'm in a bit of a career cul-de-sac. I'm 46 (no kids) and currently work in a creative role in a large company but feel increasingly under-challenged. I frequently feel that I don't have a purpose anymore, and experience lack of confidence about my abilities, which isn't helped by the fact that I'm surrounded by "fresh young talent".

I sometimes question whether I want to work in this industry at all, then other times I know I'm good at what I do, but I'm just in the wrong place to thrive. I'm so confused! I know it's never too late to change careers, but leaving my current job or taking a hefty pay cut in a new job is not an option.

Applying for jobs is quite soul-destroying as I'm competing with 30-somethings with more up-to-date skills. I'm all for extra learning and personal development, but I just feel too tired at the end of a day to do any more than I currently am doing, so I feel stuck in a rut.

MOLLY, 46

Q & A
Rachel Schofield, Career Coach and former Journalist

What are some of the common career concerns faced by midlife women?

Our careers shift into focus in different ways in midlife, but whatever our circumstances, midlife provides a natural milestone at which to stop and reflect. For some women, midlife is a moment when the career break they took to raise a family is nearing a natural end. With their children growing, they find they can come up for air again... but to do what? Head back to their old industry? Start a business? Retrain? Follow an old dream? Women in this space can often experience an unsettling combination of excitement and opportunity, coupled with self-doubt and wobbly professional identity.

For women still in work, with potentially a decade or two of employment still ahead, there's stocktaking to be done. How aligned is our career with what else is happening in life? That may be to do with the family finances, retirement plans, our partner's work, our health and wellbeing, caring for elderly parents, or our experience of the menopause.

Some women will sense it's time to slow down and broaden their focus, to scale back their work or follow a long-held dream to try something new. For others, it's finally a moment to lean into their ambitions and step up with renewed

energy and freedom. The key is to take control of the right journey for you, because there's no set blueprint for a midlife career. It's personal. I invite all my clients to get curious about who they are and what has changed over the last decade, and ask what they really want from their working life going forward.

Is it difficult to make the decision to change careers in midlife?

Our work is a major part of our identity, around which we've built a familiar structure of friendships, status, finances, routines, and even family dynamics. So, starting to move the foundations can naturally create some wobbly moments.

What's more, the human brain is hardwired to resist uncertainty. Its main concern is to keep us safe and risk-free, guiding us to stay in well-charted territory where danger is minimal and outcomes are predictable. So your brain is quick to offer you well-meaning, but often poorly evidenced, thoughts as to why a career change is impossible.

How about practical considerations?

On top of our own mind chatter come the practical challenges of making a career shift. These include things like figuring out if the new career idea is a runner, building new networks, developing fresh skills, "rebranding" ourselves, and convincing others we are a great fit.

All of these challenges require courage, commitment, and openness, and will at times cause discomfort. Career shifters have to exist for a period in a so-called "liminal space", a place of transition. The word stems from the Latin "limen", meaning threshold, and that in-between period of leaving the old but not yet feeling fully at home in the new can play temporary havoc with your sense of identity. Rest assured, that's normal.

What are the first steps towards making the leap?

A confident career shift needs three important elements and can flounder if you don't invest time in each of them. Self-reflection is an important first step, in order to build a detailed and colourful picture of yourself and the work you are after; once you've got some ideas, it's exploration time, to find answers to all of the questions and unknowns that are lurking around your favourite ideas; and when you've identified the change you want to make, the final step is transition.

We often mistakenly think a career transition is one big decision and one big move, which feels scary and often leads to paralysis. In reality, it's more often a series of many small decisions followed by a series of small but consistent actions.

How to Make a Confident Career Shift

- **Take time for self-reflection:** it's easy to charge off into the world of applications and CVs because it helps you feel like you're *doing* something. But to move forward with confidence and clarity, you first need to consider your strengths and skills. What motivates, energizes, and fulfils you? What's your definition of success? What ideas are you truly interested in? What do you need your work to look like on a practical level?

- **Explore your ideas:** from the obvious and relatively straightforward to the wild and extraordinary. Capture them all and see how they stack up against what you've outlined about what you want. Where are the good matches? How can you turn a seemingly bonkers idea into something achievable? What roles, organizations, or sectors could they lead you to?

- **Plan your transition:** how big is the gap from where you are now to where you want to be? What are the planks in the bridge you need to build? This might involve retraining, reshaping your professional network, a period in a portfolio career as you move from one thing to another, a CV and LinkedIn rewrite, re-examining your finances, and a discussion with your partner.

How can we actively create opportunities?

You can't make a career change from your sofa. People can endlessly research their career change ideas in Google, but you need to prioritize active, not passive, ways of investigating.

- Go out and talk to the people who do the work you want to do and ask them about their own career journey.
- Attend events, conferences, or workshops in person.
- Set out to get familiar with the trends, challenges, and important players in your chosen industry.
- Build relationships, knowledge, and experience by volunteering or shadowing someone.
- Run a mini project among friends to see if your dog grooming/maths tutoring/web design business could really work.

How can we build a new network?

You can't make a career change alone. Other people hold the key to your career shift and building a great new network is really important. That needn't be intimidating or formal. Start with your "warm" connections – former colleagues, friends of friends, mates from your yoga class – and approach them to connect you to people they know in your new chosen field. Just a 30-minute cup of coffee while hearing about their work can provide you with bags of valuable data. And as your confidence and clarity grows, you can reach out to people you know less well. This approach also helps you to tap into the hidden job market.

What is the "hidden job market"?

The hidden job market refers to the huge number of jobs that are never formally advertised but are filled through personal recommendation.

When you're an unusual candidate with a non-standard background, the online job application process can be slow to yield results because on paper you don't "fit". Hearing about roles that are coming up, being in the right place at the right time, having someone refer you: these are the benefits of cultivating and being active in your new network.

You can't make a career change from your sofa.

Five Ways to Upskill

1. **Look for opportunities in your current role:** apply for a secondment, ask to go on a course, volunteer for a new project, or make a side move in your existing workplace.
2. **Learn on the job:** look for a position where you can gain new skills while you are being paid, even if it's just a transitional role.
3. **Volunteer strategically:** offer to help where you'll gain valuable experience and relevant new skills.
4. **Find a mentor:** who do you know who would give you a few hours of training in that computer software you're worried about, or talk you through the transition into another field?
5. **Learn independently:** online or bite-sized courses are everywhere, meaning some skills can be acquired relatively cheaply or even for free. It's amazing what you can teach yourself with a little-and-often approach (see p.249 for resources to get you started).

How can we build self-confidence to embark on this new journey?

If your confidence is wobbly, look back over your life and career to date and build up a "confidence bank". List your strengths and skills, using lots of examples; note any achievements (professional and personal) that you're proud of; and ten things you really like about yourself.

Return to this list regularly, perhaps pin it up somewhere you'll notice it daily.

You can also try asking five people (maybe a mix of professional and personal acquaintances) to send you a list of your three top strengths and describe a time that they have experienced them.

Remember that confidence comes from taking action. If you wait to feel confident before you start, you'll be waiting a long time. Confidence is built by taking small, manageable actions that enable you to recognize what you are capable of, remind yourself of your abilities, and see what you could do to make something even better next time.

Do you have any final tips for midlife career changers?

Develop a clear narrative to explain your career journey and connect the dots between the different stages of your professional life. Look for the common threads that appear throughout, whether that's creativity, a mission to help others, a love of science, or a skillset as a communicator. Practise talking about your career shift with friends until you can describe it clearly and confidently in four or five sentences.

Your CV and LinkedIn profile shouldn't send mixed messages. Focus on where you're going, not where you've been, and ensure you adopt the keywords, language, style, and skills of your ideal new profession, not your old one.

RETURNING TO WORK AFTER A CAREER BREAK

Between the ages of 28 and 40, I took a "short" career break to bring up my four children. OK, when I say, "short break", let me assure you that it was actually 13 years of hard labour. When the youngest was finally at school full-time, I needed to find ways not only to help with the bills, but also to fill my days with something more interesting than figuring how many smiley-face frozen potato chips I should make for dinner.

But where to start and what to do? It made sense to go back to my old career of PR and marketing for a charity. A recruitment agent advised on a PR assistant role at a large social media company and I dusted off my shoulder-padded jacket for the big interview.

I felt like I had stepped into a parallel universe, where people sat on luminous green and pink chairs next to rows of purple and orange telephone boxes in a glass office. My interviewer, not much older than my eldest son, came skateboarding along the corridor to greet me.

Walking out of my very suburban home life and into this young and buzzing environment, I was filled with excitement and possibility. But equally I was scared, overwhelmed, and unsure if I could ever fit in. I know I'm not alone when it comes to feeling unconfident about how to make a career change or take the leap back into the workplace after a career break, but this can be a time of huge opportunity, and there is lots of help available to women in this situation.

I used to work in recruitment in the centre of London before having kids, but once they were old enough to go to school, I realized I wanted to find a way to work more flexibly from home so I could drop them off and pick them up each day.

After speaking to a career coach I decided to do a part-time course in social media management. It was the best decision that I ever made. It has allowed me to work from home, be there for my kids, work with so many interesting and different clients, and also – because there is no commute – make the same amount of money as I was earning in a full-time job in the city.

KATHRYN, 41

Q & A
Julianne Miles, MBE, Co-founder
and CEO of Career Returners

What is "Career Returners"?

This is a consultancy, networking, and coaching organization that I co-founded in 2014 in order to help (mainly women) professionals who'd taken long career breaks and were struggling to get back to work. We partner with over 180 employers who have created intentional routes to help get these returners back into jobs at mid- to senior levels using their professional skills and experience, or to target retraining programmes at those who've taken career breaks.

Our mission is to remove what we call the "career break penalty" – all of those challenges that make it so hard for people to get back into the workforce – and make career breaks a valued part of a lifetime career.

What are some of the most common concerns you hear from midlife women about returning to work?

What I must have heard about a thousand times is, am I employable anymore? Can I get back? Have I lost all my skills? Is anybody going to want me? Are they going to want me over a graduate? These comments all reflect the erosion of professional confidence that happens so often with many years out of a career. If you have children, you often even lose your name, introducing yourself as, "I'm so and so's mum". You can lose your sense of identity.

You may also feel disconnected from the world of work, and are not sure what you want to do or how to get back. Even for women who decide they know what they want to do, their confidence can be further knocked when they start applying for jobs through normal routes and get countless rejections or – worse – don't even hear back. They are thwarted by the recruitment biases we've been tackling since 2014.

Can you explain the recruitment biases that you've come across?

The greatest barrier for returners is the pigeonholing of candidates without recent experience as too risky to hire. This can be compounded by ageism and a false stereotype that returners aren't ambitious. We've had a lot of success in breaking down this bias, mainly within leading employers running returner programmes, but the reality is that it is still very hard for a returner to get a job via mainstream recruitment.

How can women overcome a lack of confidence about returning to work?

It's easy to focus on what a graduate has that you don't have, but when you think about what you DO have that a graduate doesn't, you start to look at it differently. You have built valuable skills before and during your career break, whatever the reason for it. Take the example of caring for children: you develop a range of skills such as time management, negotiating skills, influencing skills, and empathy. If your break is for health reasons, you build resilience and adaptability. You come back with a valuable fresh perspective, making you a stronger and better employee.

What practical things can we do?

You can begin to take steps to regain your "professional identity". Remind yourself of all your achievements and experience from before your break. Don't dismiss this as being too long ago or think that your skills are lost. I can assure you; you'll get back up to speed very quickly in the workplace. Recognize that you're just a little bit out of practice.

Get support from friends and family, asking them to give you feedback on what they think you're particularly good at. Hearing positive messages from others give you a big boost. Build a return-to-work support group with other returners so you can encourage each other.

Does fear of new technology hold a lot of us back? The idea that things have moved on without us?

You can feel that the world has changed completely in whatever sector you're in. What we hear from successful returners is that the tech may have changed, but the fundamentals of how business works remain the same. You need to get yourself back up to speed, but you are not starting from scratch.

It is worth upskilling in basic office tech to make your life easier when you are back at work and take the fear away. There are huge numbers of free courses available online (see p.249) as well as local community courses. Professional associations can be very helpful, and sometimes have free resources that can help you to upskill or conferences and events you can attend.

How important is networking?

From my experience, the majority of returners find their jobs through contacts, often friends of friends. Tell your friend that you want to get back to work and give them an idea of what you're looking for so they can introduce you to anyone

they know who could help. Take a deep breath and get back in touch with ex-colleagues, suggesting a coffee and chat. This is a great way to find out about current trends, what's changed since you left, and areas where you could update yourself. There's power in going out and talking to people and getting yourself back in the working world.

Can volunteering, while not a viable option for everyone, be one possible route back in to work?

I think it can be a good thing, but you need to be really focused on skilled volunteering. Make sure that what you are doing is going to help you to refresh or build your skills to return to work.

I am a great fan of work experience, particularly as a reality check if you're thinking about a career change or pivot. It can also be useful for finding out how things have changed if you've had a long break. I know of one returner who hadn't worked as a lawyer for 10 years who got in touch with another parent who ran a local law practice and asked if she could go in for a few mornings a week. Seeing that things actually hadn't changed that much, she was quickly contributing and ended up with a job offer.

One caveat is to limit any volunteering in the private sector. Do not spend a lot of time working for free as this undervalues what you're bringing. It's different if you want to move into the charity sector, where you often need to volunteer for a significant period before you stand a chance of getting a paid role.

Would you include a career break on your CV, or on professional platforms like LinkedIn?

I definitely would. Own your career break. Really value it. Don't apologize for it. Do not hide it. Because it's part of who you are and what you bring to an employer. This also avoids there being a mysterious break in your employment history, which could worry an employer.

LinkedIn now has a career break option, which makes this easier. It's up to you whether you want to explain the reason, such as a parental career break, a caring career break, or a health-related career break. If your break was for a painful reason that you don't want to disclose, simply put "career break". In this section, add any experience that has built your skills and experience, such as skilled volunteer work, running a small business from home, studying, living in different countries, or learning other languages.

What industries are good places to start looking?

There are lots of opportunities out there, many of which are in the tech space where they need to increase their gender diversity and they've also got big skills

Return to Work Toolkit

- Set yourself small and achievable steps and goals, such as "assess my skills" or "update my CV/résumé", and set aside time to tackle a couple of these in one go.
- Consider any ongoing caring responsibilities you may have at home, and plan how you will share out this work.
- Get into a return-to-work mindset: think about your strengths and achievements, then use your network to gather advice and boost your confidence.
- Update professional profiles such as LinkedIn, and tailor your CV for each role you apply for; emphasize your achievements and be open about your career break.
- Research the organization you are applying to in order to get a feel for what they are looking for, and prepare and practise your answers to questions before the interview.
- Don't feel you need to accept a job straight away: take time to consider what you want to discuss further or negotiate on before accepting an offer.

gaps. Other concentrations of returner employers are in financial services, professional services, and engineering. These companies recognize that women are stepping out for caring or other reasons and they're not coming back in.

Own your career
break. Really value
it. Don't apologize
for it. Do not hide it.
—

What kinds of help might be offered to welcome women returners?

Lots of companies now offer returner programmes, especially in sectors such as financial services and technology. Some of these employers now see returners as a key part of their talent strategy. The proliferation of programmes is changing attitudes more broadly towards both the longevity of careers and a recognition that careers don't always go in straight lines.

- **Returnship:** this is the most common type of programme and involves doing a job on a trial basis, giving a softer landing. We first brought the concept of returnships to the UK, but it was developed in the US and is now common practice in many sectors. You'll do a professional placement for three to six months, with a wrapper of support in the form of coaching and mentoring. Line managers also receive training in how to set up returners for success.
- **Supported hiring:** many employers offer what I call "supported hiring", which brings returners directly into permanent roles but with a similar wrapper of support, a recognition that you may need a little bit of time to get back up to speed.
- **Retraining programmes:** these target returners who are looking for a career change. These are primarily on offer in technology and finance, and they include upfront training, leading on to work opportunities.

Do you have any final words for women returning to the workforce?

I know that it can feel very isolating returning to work. Join our free Career Returners community (see p.249), or find a return-to-work support group locally to give you advice and encouragement and keep you motivated. Find role models of women who have also returned to work to build your belief that it is possible.

Be patient and persistent, as it could be a long road. But remember, a rewarding job is out there for you, and each step will get you closer to being back at work, stronger than ever.

MENOPAUSE IN THE WORKPLACE

For too long, discussion of the menopause has been taboo in the workplace. Women have suffered in silence, often counting themselves out of career progression opportunities or even quitting successful careers in order to cope. When I was in my mid-40s, I was forced to give up my career due to these symptoms. A survey by The Latte Lounge with fertility company Fertifa shows that 42% of women have considered leaving their job due to the menopause and 84% have said there is either no workplace support, or they are unsure if support exists.[1] Lost confidence, sick leave, brain fog, depression, anxiety, and fatigue can leave women feeling unable to fulfil their job demands. Menopause and perimenopause hugely impact women in the workplace.

- 14 million working days are lost in the UK because of menopause and perimenopause.[2] In the US a recent report shows that the economy loses $26.6 billion a year in lost productivity and health expenses resulting from employees managing menopause symptoms.[3]
- Three in five menopausal women say it has had a negative impact on their work, and research has shown that one in five women has left a job because of it.[4]
- One in three women wait at least three years for their symptoms to be correctly diagnosed as menopause-related, and a further 18% visit their doctor six times before they get the help they need.[5]

I'm passionate about educating women and working with employers to ensure that we get the help we need to stay in our jobs. But what happens when menopause affects your ability to do your job? As Maria Rooney's story, over the page, demonstrates, sadly, many employers do not offer adequate support for women suffering menopause symptoms and fail to understand the legal rights that

> *I loved my job working with vulnerable children and young people in care. I've been a social worker for 21 years, and studied and worked hard to get to this point. But in 2018, after 12 years' service, I was forced to resign from my job due to my menopause symptoms and my employer's conduct towards me, and had to take legal action for constructive dismissal, sex and disability discrimination, and victimization and harassment.*
>
> *I felt I had not been treated fairly and that nobody was listening to me or helping me. I submitted claims to the employment tribunal. But at a hearing in November 2019, a male judge struck out my sex and disability discrimination claims and dismissed my victimization and harassment claims. I then appealed to the Employment Appeal Tribunal (which is a high court in London) where I won all my appeals.*
>
> **MARIA, 53**

women going through the menopause may have. Maria's case established the first ever ruling by the Employment Appeal Tribunal in the UK for menopausal symptoms to be considered as a disability in relation to the Equality Act. But tribunals are a stressful, time-consuming, and expensive process.

And, unfortunately, Maria's is by no means an isolated experience. Many women have either been discriminated against or unfairly dismissed from their jobs due to their symptoms affecting their work. In fact, research from the Menopause Experts Group,[6] reveals that the number of employment tribunals citing the menopause has tripled in less than two years. So what are our employment rights when it comes to the menopause, and how can employers ensure they are doing everything possible to support and retain their valuable talent?

Q & A
Michael Kerrigan, Employment Law Specialist
and Partner at Debenhams Ottaway Solicitors

Why has menopause become a legal issue?

I'm an employment lawyer with over 15 years' experience advising employers and employees, but it is only in the last three to four years that I have been asked to provide any advice on the menopause. This coincided with the explosion of coverage in the media and a surge in public interest on this topic. I was shocked by the stories that I was hearing and about how, historically, employers had made little to no effort to understand the menopause or seek to support women.

What should women do if they are struggling with menopause in the workplace?

They should inform their employer in writing, highlight any aspect of their employment that is causing them difficulties, and propose adjustments that may help. Women should consider what support from their employer is reasonable: this will be viewed against a number of factors including the cost, the resources of the employer, and the disruption that the adjustment may have on the business.

Women should enquire if their employer has any existing menopause policy, a useful first port of call to establish what assistance and support may be on offer. Employers may request input from third parties, including occupational health specialists, to advise on what adjustments may be appropriate for specific symptoms.

What if there is no improvement, following these actions?

I would hope that when an employee raises concerns at an early stage, their employer would work with them to offer support and avoid the situation escalating. If, having expressly informed their employer, there is a failure to implement any adjustments or if any other discriminatory treatment related to menopause occurs, the employee is more likely to be able to undermine any defence from the employer that they simply didn't know of the symptoms.

Women should be mindful of their right to raise formal grievances if they are unhappy about any aspect of their employment and how they are being treated at work. This will normally trigger a formal process during which the employee has an opportunity to raise their complaints in a formal setting, which then require a formal response from the employer and provide a right of appeal.

What practical things can an employer put in place to help?

Once an employer becomes aware of an employee's disability, British law states there is an obligation under the Equality Act 2010 for them to make changes to remove or reduce a disadvantage that an employee is suffering due to a disability.

Employment tribunals are increasingly willing to find that menopause symptoms such as insomnia, brain fog, and anxiety can amount to a disability under the Equality Act and trigger the obligation for employers to provide what are known as "reasonable adjustments". These changes will often be very specific to an individual employee's job and their needs, involving measures including:

- physical changes to a workplace (e.g. installing a ramp for wheelchair access)
- changing someone's working pattern (e.g. allowing more flexible working hours)
- providing equipment (e.g. a specialist keyboard or chair)

Reasonable adjustments could be as simple as providing a fan to counteract the effect of hot flushes, or be more impactful, such as allowing regular short breaks or flexible working times to deal with lack of sleep due to insomnia or night sweats.

Good Menopause Practice in the Workplace

- Specialist training for internal menopause champions who will support impacted employees on the ground
- Hybrid and flexible working across the business
- Offering private areas for women to rest or access personal or professional support
- Dress code: offering a choice of breathable fabric and menopause-friendly designs for staff uniforms

How can women raise a formal grievance and/or take legal action?

With discrimination claims, the employee bringing a claim will need to demonstrate that the treatment complained of was because of a characteristic that is protected by the Equality Act 2010 and not for another non-discriminatory reason. The employee will therefore need to show that the employer knew they were disabled when the alleged discrimination occurred. In view of the complexity and evolving nature of employment law, I recommend that anyone considering raising a formal grievance or pursuing legal action against their employer seeks specialist legal advice first.

"

When I was struggling at work, due to being constantly exhausted from dealing with night sweats, I asked my manager if I would be able to work more flexibly, with more days working from home and later starts after a bad night.

They were not only willing to help find a way to accommodate my requests, but have also asked me to be a "menopause champion", organizing monthly meet-ups where women support and share stories with each other and get advice from different specialists on how to cope with menopause symptoms at home and at work.

ESTHER, 56

What are the benefits to employers in supporting women dealing with menopause?

Employers who do engage on this issue are likely to reap the rewards. It makes economic sense for employers to commit to supporting women through menopause. Firstly for selfish reasons, to avoid potentially costly legal claims, but also to ensure that they are able to harness a wealth of experience and knowledge from female members of staff who may previously have been forced to end their careers early due to menopause.

What does the future look like in terms of menopause support in the workplace?

We have seen a huge amount of progress in removing the stigma around menopause in recent years, and HRT is even being paid for by some forward-thinking employers where it has been prescribed. But it is very important that we try to maintain the current momentum around this issue to ensure that legal protections for women going through menopause become as central to our thinking as maternity rights and flexible working.

Finance

Lots of us might feel out of our depth, confused, or scared when it comes to understanding and managing our finances. It can be hard to know when and how to plan for a comfortable financial future, with the ever-rising cost of living forcing so many of us to work harder and for longer than ever before. But quite often, like so many things in life, the fear is far worse than the reality. With the right help and planning, we can confidently step into a happier and more secure future.

MONEY MANAGEMENT

One of the most important lessons I've learnt from running The Latte Lounge is to surround yourself with people who know far more than you in any area that you don't understand. I've also learnt to never be afraid to ask if you don't understand something. Mastering money management can be truly empowering, and there are some simple tools that will allow you to stay on top of your finances by creating habits that will help you to plan for financial security.

The debt crisis worldwide continues to grow year on year, with many living pay check to pay check, struggling to manage, or taking on debt at an alarming rate. The financial pressures for everyone are considerable: food, bills, childcare, commuting, large mortgage costs. On top of this, the retirement age has risen, and pension arrangements have changed, so many of us are having to find extra money to put towards retirement.

Nobody teaches us at school or university about the importance of managing our finances or planning for the future, but one of the biggest things you can do to reduce stress around money is to become educated about it. There are lots of great resources available to help you become more organized with your savings, outgoings, and paperwork too (see p.249).

I have never been very good at planning for the future or saving, because pretty much all of my income (as a single mum) goes straight back out to pay for the mortgage, food, kids' stuff, holidays, and utility bills. I've been worried recently about the future, so I decided to speak to a Financial Advisor.

One of the best pieces of advice she gave me was that the only way to be successful with saving is to make it a habit. Ever since then I have set up automated small monthly deposits going into a separate savings account so I can "set it and forget it", as she put it. Why, oh why, didn't I think of that 20 years ago!'

CASSIE, 43

Q & A
Eileen Adamson, Money Coach

What should we be thinking about with regard to our finances post 40?

As we step into our 40s and beyond, it's crucial to have a clear understanding of our current financial situation and think about future planning. It's time to get rid of financial fear and instead embrace money matters with confidence and a feeling of empowerment.

Focus on the three Fs: Freedom, Flexibility, and Fun. Financial freedom is not just about accumulating wealth, it's also about gaining control over our financial future: whether that's the freedom for a career change, a dream holiday, or even early retirement. Money isn't only about bills and responsibilities; it's also a ticket to enjoy life and create memorable experiences.

Becoming curious about money allows us to make informed decisions. We are not just capable of handling our finances, we are also capable of mastering them.

How can we get a handle on our financial situation?

Assess your income, expenses, liabilities, and savings. Make sure you have a budget in place and stick to it. It's not just about cutting costs; it's about making your money work for you. It's equally important

to actively contribute towards your retirement fund, consider potential healthcare costs, and account for inflation.

Financial planning isn't a one-time activity, it's a continuous process that requires regular reviews and adjustments as your life circumstances and financial goals change. Educate yourself, be proactive in your financial management, and don't hesitate to seek professional advice if you need it. Do a money makeover (see opposite); this will help make your money work in alignment with your values and long-term goals.

What common financial concerns do you hear from midlife women?

Many fear making mistakes that might jeopardize their financial stability or retirement plans. Inaction is often a consequence of this, as it seems easier to ignore it than potentially get it wrong.

A mistake that many women make is not investing due to a fear of risk. Understandably, the volatility of the market can seem daunting; however, keeping all your money in a savings account, where inflation can erode its value, is not ideal either. Spreading the money across different pots and understanding your personal tolerance to risk can help mitigate potential losses.

Money Makeover

1. Print out statements (bank statements, credit card, etc.) from the past month.

2. Grab three coloured pens and categorize all your expenses into needs (e.g. bills), wants (such as entertainment and holidays), and savings contributions/debt repayments.

3. Calculate what percentage of your income is spent in each of the three areas. Ideally you should spend no more than 50% on needs and 30% on wants, with 20% going into savings.

4. Identify what's most important to you: it may be health, family, career, travel, or giving back to the community.

5. Examine your spending from the past month. Is it in alignment with these values? If not, consider ways you can adjust your spending to better reflect what truly matters to you.

6. Create a 50/30/20 values-based spending plan for the future. Prioritize spending on the things that matter the most: e.g. if fitness is a top value, a larger portion of your "wants" budget might go towards a gym membership.

Some midlife women are concerned about the expense of helping their children as they turn into young adults: driving lessons, university costs, and first home. Having little or no savings is another issue for many, and unexpected costs can completely disrupt their financial security.

Where can we go when we need more support with managing our finances?

If you're looking to build your financial confidence or improve your relationship with money, a Financial Coach might be the answer. They'll help you to understand your financial habits, define your values, and align your spending to match those values, turning money management into a positive – rather than stressful – part of life. Find certified coaches at the Association for Coaching (see p.249).

For more detailed advice on financial planning, a Financial Advisor can be a great asset. They can clarify your current financial situation, help set achievable goals, and map out a plan for you to reach them. Find certified advisors via the Financial Conduct Authority (see p.249).

Enlisting the help of professionals can be a real game-changer. These experts can equip you with the tools to take command of your finances, laying the groundwork for a secure financial future. Take a deep breath, and know that there are people there to help you every step of the way.

What advice can you offer to those of us struggling with managing debt?

When women are struggling to manage their money on a day-to-day basis, they can often end up burying their head in the sand. Subsequently, this avoidance tends to result in a build-up of debt, whether it's from credit cards, loans, or unpaid bills.

As the debt accumulates, the financial pressure increases, leading to a vicious cycle of avoidance and escalating debt.

Even if debt is not an issue, money can be easily wasted each month, which would be better used in planning for retirement or investing in your own health and happiness. Ignoring financial problems seldom makes them disappear; instead, it exacerbates them. It's never too late to change financial habits. It's about shifting from a reactive to a proactive strategy, where you have control over your finances, and not the other way around.

For advice in handling debt, StepChange is a wonderful resource (see p.249). This UK-based debt charity offers free, expert advice to help you deal with your debts, and provides solutions tailored to your individual circumstances, allowing you to repay your debts in a manageable way.

How prepared are most of us for retirement?

One of the most frequently voiced fears I hear is of being unprepared for retirement, often alongside the worry of not having enough savings to sustain a comfortable lifestyle. Many women will admit that they don't understand pensions, don't understand how to plan for retirement, and are terrified of not knowing how to solve this problem.

With women generally outliving men, it's essential that we prepare for a longer retirement period. This means saving more and planning for potential healthcare expenses in later life. Some women can neglect their pension schemes, particularly if they've taken career breaks to raise a family or care for loved ones. It's vital to consider the long-term impact on pension savings and explore options to make up for the lost time.

Many women also underestimate the cost of retirement, failing to factor in inflation and unexpected expenses, such as additional health and care costs as they age. Accurate forecasting is the key to a secure retirement. There are loads of great online resources that can help with the process of calculating retirement costs for different scenarios (see p.249).

How can we make sure we are planning sufficiently for the future?

First establish a clear timeline of estimated expenses from now until retirement. This should include routine expenses, potential healthcare costs, lifestyle expenses, and any other costs that are likely to arise. Each of these should be evaluated and a potential cost assigned to them.

To do this, tools like financial calculators budgeting apps, or professional financial planning services can be invaluable. It's not just about surviving retirement, but enjoying it! Think about your retirement lifestyle and plan accordingly. Once you have an idea of the total cost over the years, you can start planning how you will meet these expenses.

It's not just about surviving retirement, but enjoying it! Think about your retirement lifestyle and plan accordingly.

—

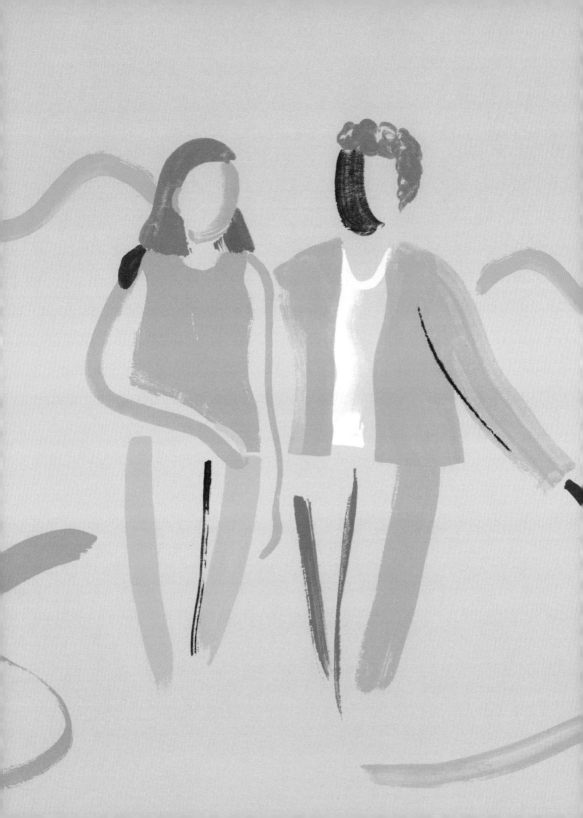

Andrea McLean,
Broadcaster, Author, and Coach

REINVENTION

When we reach midlife, we often assess our lives and feel like something needs to change, whether this has to do with our career goals, our health and wellbeing, or within our personal relationships. And when you decide you want to make a change to your life, it's more often than not something that has been bubbling away for a long time. It may seem to come out of the blue, but it's actually a thought, feeling, or desire that's been percolating, growing stronger over time.

And then there comes the pivot point where you ask yourself: "Am I going to keep thinking about this as an idea or a dream, or am I actually going to do something about it? Am I going to step off this ledge into the unknown, or am I going to stay here, where it feels uncomfortable but familiar, too scared to try?" The biggest mistake that women make when it comes to making changes in their lives is waiting until everything is "just right" before taking any kind of action. Spoiler alert: there is never a perfect time. Ever.

Everyone talks about building a blueprint for success, but what's really important is building a blueprint for failure: work out as much as possible what you will do if everything goes wrong – as well as planning for the things that you want to go right.

If you are feeling stuck, the first thing I'd say to you is acknowledge it. Acknowledge what your body and your brain are trying to tell you. It may feel like anxiety, or a rumbling sense that things aren't quite right. Headaches, teeth clenching, and churning stomach: these are often signs that your body is trying to tell you that something is not as it should be, and you are stuck in a place that you don't want to be in.

My advice is to get a notebook, or use the Notes section of your phone, and start writing down how you would like your life to be. Start writing it down now. If you don't know where to start, then write down what you don't like. We tend to find this much easier to do, and it's really easy to flip it 180 degrees: I don't want that = I want this.

Before you know it, you have a plan. You have a series of goals that you can work towards, and the minute you start working towards a goal, you're not looking at the problem anymore, you're looking at the solution. And this is where it gets really exciting!

When you start looking at the solution, it's like doors open, like you can see the road ahead. This instantly helps you to feel better, even if nothing has actually changed yet. How? Because you are looking at things differently. You're thinking differently. This is how you come unstuck, and this is how change begins.

A LETTER TO ALL MIDLIFE WOMEN

I hope that, having reached the end of this book, you will be feeling more empowered and excited about the possibilities that this next chapter of life can bring and how you want your life to pan out moving forward.

Midlife is a time of soul searching and discovery: it's for discovering the things that matter to you most, deciding what doesn't matter anymore, and considering what you can do to shake things up to ensure a happier, healthier, and more fulfilled second chapter.

Amid the many demands of midlife, it's so important to focus on your needs and desires and not just those of others. Self-care is not selfish, it's vital to ensure that we are not only there for those that rely on us, but that we can show up for ourselves too, that we matter and deserve to experience joy.

Whatever your situation, try not to think of these years as a "midlife crisis", but more a time of "midlife reinvention".

You might revisit dreams, aspirations, and passions you had in your younger years; perhaps you'll search for a new relationship; maybe you're ready to re-train and embark on a new career, or an adventure?

It's taken me nearly half a century to get here, but I feel like I'm finally free to be my true self and live the life I was meant to live. I wanted to write this book so that I could help you to feel this way too, by sharing everything I have learnt from my own personal experiences, but also by bringing together some of the world's leading experts to share their knowledge and expertise. In some ways, I've written the book that I wish I had been given as a 40th birthday gift to keep by my bed, one that would guide me over the many bumps I've experienced.

Remember that knowledge is power, and change takes time. But if you can learn to advocate confidently for yourself and make small and steady changes, it will help to make this journey through midlife and beyond so much smoother and more enjoyable.

You are not alone, and we are stronger together, so surround yourself with other like-minded women and lean on each other when times get tough, but please don't forget to also celebrate all the wins and good times together too, because life is short and precious, and midlife can be such an exciting and liberating time.

All that's left to say is thank you for reading, and go live life to the full!

Lots of love and lattes,

Katie xxx

TESTIMONIALS

"Katie is a pioneer for better support and awareness for women in menopause, sharing her own experiences as well as those of The Latte Lounge community to start important conversations around midlife health and wellbeing."

Trish Halpin & Lorraine Candy, hosts of the Postcards from Midlife podcast

....

"Katie is a tireless campaigner who has been at the forefront of the menopause movement for the last nine years. Her work, through both the Latte Lounge and The Midlife Festival, has provided a vital platform for women's menopause stories to be heard, as well as helping to fill in the huge gaps that still persist in menopause awareness and education."

Sarah Graham, journalist and author of Rebel Bodies

....

"My daughter, Katie Taylor, decided to use her own experience to help other women navigate midlife more easily. Via The Latte Lounge platform that she founded nine years ago, she has been supporting, educating, and signposting women, and campaigning for better menopause and women's health support."

Professor Michael Baum, Emeritus Professor of Surgery, UCL

....

"Katie has dedicated her life to supporting women through the perimenopause and menopause, as well as campaigning for change and educating companies about how to support their employees. Katie is the supportive friend you'd want by your side throughout midlife, signposting and encouraging you at every step."

Anna O'Sullivan, co-founder of The Midlife Festival

....

"Katie has been a trusted voice and powerhouse in the menopause space for almost a decade. She has dedicated herself to providing women with quality information to help them through menopause and beyond."

Fiona Clark, Director of Harley Street Emporium

....

"I have known Katie for years, having worked with her on a number of menopause projects including a talk at number 10 Downing Street to discuss menopause in the workplace. She has always been passionate about supporting women going through the menopause and a strong supporter of having accurate information available to guide women."

Mr Haitham Hamoda MD FRCOG, Consultant Gynaecologist and clinical lead for The Menopause Service, Kings

NOTES

SECTION 1: HEALTH

1   thebms.org.uk/wp-content/uploads/2023/06/20-BMS-TfC-Menopause-in-ethnic-minority-women-JUNE2023-A.pdf
2   www.ncbi.nlm.nih.gov/pmc/articles/PMC5415400
3   www.ons.gov.uk/peoplepopulationandcommunity/birthsdeathsandmarriages/deaths/bulletins/suicidesintheunitedkingdom/2021registrations#suicide-patterns-by-age
4   www.nice.org.uk/guidance/NG23
5   www.cambridge.org/core/journals/bjpsych-bulletin/article/severe-mental-illness-and-the-perimenopause/8D072AACBCD3C7888C173B36635C08C3
6   British Menopause Society, see note 1
7   legacy.synergicollaborativecentre.co.uk/wp-content/uploads/2017/11/Synergi_Report_Web.pdf
8   British Menopause Society, see note 1
9   Brown JP, et al. 2009. Relations among menopausal symptoms, sleep disturbance and depressive symptoms in midlife. pubmed.ncbi.nlm.nih.gov/19128903
10 Timur S, Sahin NH. 2010. Prevalence of depression and influencing factors in perimenopausal & postmenopausal women. pubmed.ncbi.nlm.nih.gov/20400922
11 add.org/adhd-questionnaire
12 www.fertifa.com/post/menopause-survey
13 www.reproductivefacts.org/globalassets/_rf/news-and-publications/booklets/fact-sheets/english-pdf/Age_and_Fertility.pdf
14 eveappeal.org.uk/gynaecological-cancers
15 eveappeal.org.uk/gynaecological-cancers/womb-cancer
16 eveappeal.org.uk/gynaecological-cancers/vaginal-cancer
17 nhsjewishbrcaprogramme.org.uk
18 www.who.int/news-room/fact-sheets/detail/breast-cancer
19 www.cancerresearchuk.org/health-professional/cancer-statistics/statistics-by-cancer-type/breast-cancer/mortality#heading-Two
20 Marmot MG, Altman DG, Cameron DA, et al. 2013. The benefits and harms of breast cancer screening pubmed.ncbi.nlm.nih.gov/23744281
21 www.cancer.org/cancer/types/breast-cancer/risk-and-prevention/breast-cancer-risk-factors-you-cannot-change.html
22 Marmot MG, Altman DG, Cameron DA, et al, see note 20
23 Mittra I, Mishra GA, Dikshit RP et al. 2021. Effect of screening by clinical breast examination on breast cancerincidence & mortality after 20 years www.ncbi.nlm.nih.gov/pmc/articles/PMC7903383
24 gettingitrightfirsttime.co.uk/wp-content/uploads/2021/09/BreastSurgeryReport-Jul21p.pdf
25 www.targit.org.uk
26 www.cancer.org/cancer/types/breast-cancer/risk-and-prevention/breast-cancer-risk-factors-you-cannot-change.html
27 breast.predict.cam/tool
28 www.bhf.org.uk/-/media/files/for-professionals/research/heart-statistics/bhf-cvd-statistics-uk-factsheet.pdf
29 Maas AH, Franke HR. Women's health in menopause with a focus on hypertension. Neth Heart J. 2009. pubmed.ncbi.nlm.nih.gov/19247469
30 Sciomer S, Moscucci F, Salvioni E, Marchese G, Bussotti M, Corrà U, Piepoli MF. Role of gender, age and BMI in prognosis of heart failure. Eur J Prev Cardiol. 2020. pubmed.ncbi.nlm.nih.gov/33238736
31 Landy, R, Pesola, F, Castañón, A, et al. 2016. Impact of cervical screening on cervical cancer mortality. pubmed.ncbi.nlm.nih.gov/27632376/
32 www.cochrane.org/CD001877/BREASTCA_screening-for-breast-cancer-with-mammography

SECTION 2: WELLBEING

1   www.bonehealthandosteoporosis.org/preventing-fractures/general-facts/what-women-need-to-know
2   bjsm.bmj.com/content/57/20/1317
3   pubmed.ncbi.nlm.nih.gov/30098758
4   academic.oup.com/cercor/article/27/8/4083/3056452

SECTION 3: PERSONAL LIFE

1   www.ons.gov.uk/peoplepopulationandcommunity/populationandmigration/populationestimates
2   Reis, H T, Regan, A, & Lyubomirsky, S. 2021. Interpersonal chemistry. journals.sagepub.com/doi/abs/10.1177/1745691621994241
3   Dr Anna Machin, Why We Love, W&N, 2022
4   cherwell.org/2024/02/07/friendships-dunbar-number
5   www.carersuk.org/reports/valuing-carers-research-report
6   www.carersuk.org/policy-and-research/key-facts-and-figures

SECTION 4: WORK & FINANCE

1   www.fertifa.com/post/menopause-survey
2   Survey of 1,000 women over 50, commissioned by Health & Her, carried out by Censuswide, March 2019. Supplementing the research are official figures from the Office of National Statistics which show that there are 4,357,000 working women aged 50–64 in the UK.
3   time.com/6274622/menopause-us-economy-women-work
4   Research by CIPD, the professional body for HR and people development www.cipd.org/uk/about/press-releases/menopause-at-work
5   Survey of 5,000 women conducted by Newson Health Research and Education found that a third of women wait at least three years for their symptoms to be correctly diagnosed as menopause-related, and a further 18% visited their doctor six times before they got the right help.
6   menopauseexperts.com/tribunals-triple-in-less-than-2-years

RESOURCES

These resources are organized by topic: some are referenced in the relevant chapter, but there are also additional resources that we hope you will find helpful. As your first port of call, please visit Katie's Latte Lounge website, where you will find a wealth of advice and information on all of the issues within the book, plus the opportunity to engage with a truly supportive community.

www.lattelounge.co.uk

SECTION 1: HEALTH

MENOPAUSE

Websites:
Australasian Menopause Society: www.menopause.org.au
British Menopause Society: www.thebms.org.uk
Canadian Menopause Society: www.sigmamenopause.com
European Menopause and Andropause Society: www.emas-online.org
Harley Street at Home: www.harleystathome.com
Indian Menopause Society: indianmenopausesociety.org
The Menopause Charity: www.themenopausecharity.org
Menopause Support: www.menopausesupport.co.uk
Nick Panay private practice: www.hormonehealth.co.uk
North American Menopause Society: www.menopause.org
Queer Menopause: www. queermenopause.com
South African Menopause Society: www.menopause.co.za

Books:
Bluming, Dr Avrum & Carol Tavris, *Oestrogen Matters*, revised edition, Little, Brown, 2024
Danzebrink, Diane, *Making Menopause Matter*, Sheldon Press, 2024
Fadal, Tamsen, *How to Menopause*, Hachette Go, 2025

Earle, Liz, *A Better Second Half*, Yellow Kite, 2024
Frostrup, Mariella & Alice Smellie, *Cracking The Menopause*, Bluebird, 2022
Harper, Dr Shahzadi & Emma Bardwell, *The Perimenopause Solution: Take control of your hormones before they take control of you*, Vermilion, 2021
Kaye, Dr Philippa, *The M Word: Everything you need to know about the menopause*, Hachette, 2023
Kaye, Dr Philippa, *The Science of the Menopause*, DK, 2024
McCall, Davina & Dr Naomi Potter, Menopausing, new edition, HQ, 2024
McLean, Andrea, *Confessions of a Menopausal Woman*, Bantam Press, 2018
Short, Hannah & Dr Mandy Leonhardt, *The Complete Guide to POI & Early Menopause*, Sheldon Press, 2022

Podcasts:
The Latte Lounge, Midlife and Menopause Uncovered: podcasts.apple.com/us/podcast/the-latte-lounge-podcast/id1626848207
The Happy Hormones Podcast: podcasts.apple.com/us/podcast/happy-hormones-podcast/id1497554597
The Happy Menopause Podcast: podcasts.apple.com/us/podcast/the-happy-menopause/id1468784256
Menopause and Cancer: podcasts.apple.com/gb/podcast/the-menopause-and-cancer- podcast/id1631842514
Menopause Whilst Black: podcasts. apple.com/gb/podcast/menopause-whilst-black/id1537012198

MENTAL & BRAIN HEALTH

Websites:
Attention Deficit Disorder Association: add.org/adhd-test
ADHD, Kate Moryoussef: www.adhdwomenswellbeing.co.uk
B-eat (eating disorder charity): www.beateatingdisorders.org.uk
David Gittleston, Psychotherapist, The Green Door Practice: www.gittelson.net
Dr Emma Ping, GP specializing in menopause and ADHD:

www.menopausecare.co.uk
Guy Leschziner, Consultant Neurologist: www.guyleschziner.com
Dr Philippa Kaye, GP: www.drphilippakaye.com
Dr Sophie Behrman, Consultant Psychiatrist: www.oxfordhealth.nhs.uk
Dr Wendy Molefi, GP & Menopause Specialist: www.vitalwellnessclinic.com
National Autistic Society: www.autism.org.uk
NHS Talking Therapies: www.nhs.uk
Samaritans (mental health helpline): 116 123 www.samaritans.org

REPRODUCTIVE & PELVIC HEALTH

Websites:
Prof Dame Lesley Regan DBE, clinics: www.onewelbeck.com and NHS clinic at www.imperial.nhs.uk
Endometriosis UK: www.endometriosis-uk.org
Gidon Lieberman, Gynaecologist: www.mrgidonlieberman.co.uk
IAPMD (International Association for Premenstrual Disorders www.iapmd.org
Kym Vopni, Pelvic Health Physiotherapist: www.vaginacoach.com
NAPS (National Association for Pre-menstrual Syndromes): www.pms.org.uk
Wellbeing of Women: www.wellbeingofwomen.org.uk

Apps:
NHS Squeezy: squeezyapp.com

Books:
Simpson, Jane, *The Pelvic Floor Bible*, Penguin Life, 2019
Vopni, Kym, *Your Pelvic Floor*, Watkins Publishing, 2021

GYNAE & BREAST CANCERS

Websites:
Breast Cancer Now: breastcancernow.org
The Eve Appeal: eveappeal.org.uk
Prof Jayant Vaidya, Professor of Surgery and Oncology: www.jayantvaidya.org
Macmillan Cancer Support: www.macmillan.org.uk
NHS: www.nhs.uk/conditions/breast-screening-mammogram

Books:
Baum, Prof Michael, *The History & Mystery of Breast Cancer*, Cambridge Scholars Publishing, 2022
Vaidya, Jayant S & Vivek Patkar, *Fast Facts: Early Breast Cancer*, Karger, 2023

HEART HEALTH

Websites:
Dr Amanda Varnava, Cardiologist: www.amandavarnava.co.uk

MUSCULOSKELETAL HEALTH

Websites:
Prof Hasan Tahir, Consultant Rheumatologist: www.hasantahir.com

SECTION 2: WELLBEING

Websites:
NHS Live Well: www.nhs.uk/live-well

DIET & NUTRITION

Websites:
Jackie Lynch, Nutritionist: www.well-well-well.co.uk
Sophie Medlin, Dietitian: www.citydietitians.co.uk

Books:
Lynch, Jackie, *The Happy Menopause, Smart Nutrition to Help You Flourish*, Watkins Publishing, 2020
Williams, Nicki, *It's Not You, It's Your Hormones*, Practical Inspiration Publishing, 2017

FITNESS

Websites:
Dinah Siman, Menopause Pilates: www.menopausepilates.com
Kate Oakley, Your Future Fit: www.yourfuturefit.com
Petra Coveney: www.menopause-yoga.com

Books:
Minchin, Louise, *Fearless: Adventures With Extraordinary Women*, Bloomsbury, 2023
Thebe, Amanda, *Menopocalypse: How I learned to thrive during menopause and how you can too*, Greystone Books, 2020

Rowe-Ham, Kate, *Owning Your Menopause: Fitter, Calmer, Stronger in 30 Days*, Yellow Kite, 2023
Mehta, Lavina MBE, *The Feel Good Fix: Boost Energy, Improve Sleep and Move More Through Menopause and Beyond*, Penguin Life, 2024

SLEEP

Websites:
Prof Guy Leschziner, Consultant Neurologist: www.guyleschziner.com
Marianne Taylor: www.thesleepworks.co.uk

Books:
Leschziner, Prof Guy, *The Secret World of Sleep: Tales of Nightmares and Neuroscience*, Simon & Schuster, 2019

RESTORING CALM

Websites:
Natasha Harris, Mindfulness and Wellbeing Coach: www.mindbodysoulenergy.co.uk
Professional Standards Authority: www.professionalstandards.org.uk
Sally Garozzo, Clinical Hypnotherapist: www.sallygarozzo.com

Podcasts:
The Menopause Mindset: podcasts.apple.com/gb/podcast/the-menopause-mindset/id1506366775

Apps:
Calm www.calm.com
Headspace www.headspace.com

SELF-CARE

Websites:
Dr Amiee Vyas, Practitioner in Aesthetic Medicine: www.doctoramiee.com
Gayle Rinkoff, Fashion and Celebrity Stylist: www.gaylerinkoff.com
Dr Hélène du P. Menagé, Consultant Dermatologist: www.onewelbeck.com
Michael Douglas, Celebrity Hairdresser: www.mdlondon.co.uk
Michelle Griffith Robinson, Life Coach: www.michellegriffithrobinsonoly.co.uk
Ruby Hammer MBE, Makeup Artist: www.rubyhammer.com

SECTION 3: PERSONAL LIFE

SEX & RELATIONSHIPS

Websites:
The Blue Ticks, relationship coaching: www.theblueticks.com
Dr Shahzadi Harper, GP specializing in womens health: www.theharperclinic.com
Tamsen Fadal, journalist and menopause advocate: www.tamsenfadal.com

Books:
Fadal, Tamsen, *The New Single: Finding, Fixing, and Falling Back in Love with Yourself After a Breakup or Divorce*, St Martins Press, 2015
McLean, Andrea, *This Girl Is On Fire*, Hay House, 2020
Wilby, Rosie, *The Breakup Monologues: The Unexpected Joy of Heartbreak*, Green Tree, 2023

PARTNERSHIP PROBLEMS

Websites:
Caron Barruw, Psychotherapist: www.caronbarruw.org
Neil Russell, Head of the Family Dept at Seddons Solicitors: www.seddons.co.uk

FRIENDSHIPS

Websites:
Claire Cohen, Journalist: clairecohen.substack.com

Books:
Cohen, Claire, *BFF? The truth about female friendship*, Penguin, 2023

Podcasts:
BFF? With Claire Cohen: podcasts.apple.com/us/podcast/bff-with-claire-cohen/id1628638433

FAMILY MATTERS

Websites:
Age UK (advice on supporting older people): www.ageuk.org.uk
Angels Support (autism and ADHD support for families): angelssupportgroup.org.uk
Care Home (UK independent reviews): www.carehome.co.uk CarersUK.org

Carers UK (support and practical advice for carers in the UK): www.carersuk.org
Childline: 0800 1111 www.childline.org.uk
Dementia UK (support for those affected by dementia): www.dementiauk.org
Home Care (independent reviews of UK elder care): www.homecare.co.uk
Jackie Gray, The Carents Room: www.carents.co.uk
Leanne Cowan, Chartered Clinical Psychologist: www.kindlekids.org.uk
MindEd (free educational resource on children, young people, adults, and older people's mental health): www.minded.org.uk
The Mix (support for under 25s): www.themix.org.uk
National Bullying Helpline: www.nationalbullyinghelpline.co.uk
NSPCC: www.nspcc.org.uk
Student Minds (mental health charity for students): www.studentminds.org.uk
Young Minds: www.youngminds.org.uk/parent

National care regulators:
England: The Care Quality Commission (CQC) cqc.org.uk
Northern Ireland: The Regulation and Quality Improvement Authority (RQIA) www.rqia.org.uk
Scotland: The Care Inspectorate (CIS) www.careinspectorate.com
Wales: The Care Inspectorate (CIW) careinspectorate.wales

Books:
Candy, Lorraine, *'Mum, What's Wrong with You?': 101 Things Only Mothers of Teenage Girls Know*, Fourth Estate, 2021

GRIEF

Websites:
Dr Shelley Gilbert MBE (PHD) PGDPM, PGDC, Cert in Clinical Supervision, Snr Accredited MBACP, UKRCP Reg. www.thegriefdoctor.co.uk
Grief Encounter (bereavement charity founded by Dr Shelley Gilbert): www.griefencounter.org.uk
Apart of Me (charity supporting bereaved children, young people, and parents): apartofme.app

Child Bereavement UK (helps children and families when a child dies or is grieving): www.childbereavementuk.org
Cruse Bereavement Care (charity for bereaved people in England, Wales, & Northern Ireland): www.cruse.org.uk
Widowed and Young (charity for people aged 50 or under whose partner has died): www.widowedandyoung.org.uk

SECTION 4: WORK & FINANCE

WORK

Websites:
Julianne Miles MBE, CEO of Career Returners: careerreturners.com
Michael Kerrigan, Employment Law Specialist at Debenhams Ottaway: www.debenhamsottaway.co.uk
Rachel Schofield, Career Coach: www.rachelschofield.co.uk
Advisory, Conciliation and Arbitration Service (ACAS): www.acas.org.uk/menopause-at-work

Books:
Miles, Julianne, *Second Act*, Piatkus Books, 2025
Schofield, Rachel, *The Career Change Guide: Five steps to finding your dream job*, Michael Joseph, 2023

Upskilling:
Alison (free online accredited vocational courses): alison.com
LinkedIn Learning (guided learning in business, creative, and technology skills): www.linkedin.com/learning
Coursera (online accredited courses): coursera.org
Udemy (online courses in professional development): www.udemy.com
Women to Work (coaching and programmes to support women in the workplace): www.womentowork.co.uk
YouTube (for free, bite-sized information videos on a wide range of subjects)

FINANCES

Websites:
Eileen Adamson, Money Coach: www.yourmoneysorted.co.uk

Budget Planner (free money-management tool): www.moneysavingexpert.com
Association for Coaching (help finding a financial coach): www.associationforcoaching.com
Retirement Living Standards (help in planning for retirement): www.retirementlivingstandards.org.uk
StepChange (UK-based debt charity offering free, expert advice): www.stepchange.org
The Financial Conduct Authority (financial advice plus UK directory of registered firms and advisors): www.fca.org.uk

GENERAL SUPPORT

Addiction Helper (information and resources for anyone who is affected by addiction): www.addictionhelper.com
Citizens Advice (free practical advice on everything from debt to health and legal matters): www.citizensadvice.org.uk
Counselling Directory (find verified professional therapists in the UK): www.counselling-directory.org.uk
Give Us a Shout (text Shout to 85258. Free, confidential, 24/7 text messaging support service for anyone struggling to cope): www.giveusashout.org
My Pickle (help and support on a range of topics in the UK): www.mypickle.org
Refuge (UK helpline supporting women and children fleeing domestic abuse): 0808 2000 247 www.nationaldahelpline.org.uk
Rape Crisis (help for women, with 38 Rape Crisis Centres across England and Wales): www.rapecrisis.org.uk
Rights of Women (free legal advice and information for women experiencing violence): www.rightsofwomen.org.uk
Samaritans (mental health helpline): 116 123 www.samaritans.org
Talk To Frank (facts and support on drugs and alcohol): www.talktofrank.com
With You (free, confidential support for anyone experiencing issues with addiction or mental health): www.wearewithyou.org.uk
Women's Aid (UK charity working to end domestic abuse against women and children): www.womensaid.org.uk

INDEX

KATIE TAYLOR

Katie Taylor is the founder and CEO of The Latte Lounge, an online platform for women over 40, which exists to help women in midlife thrive at home and in the workplace. She hosts a variety of events, including "The Midlife Festival" and The Latte Lounge podcast, "Midlife and Menopause Uncovered".

Katie offers a consultancy service for organizations who want to help women with menopause support in the workplace – a professional highlight included running a "Menopause in the Workplace" awareness event for all the staff at No 10 Downing Street.

Katie has proudly campaigned for years alongside the #MakeMenopauseMatter team, founded by Diane Danzebrink, to help ensure that menopause is added to the UK secondary school and medical school curriculums and included in workplace policies. She has provided evidence to the government to ensure that menopause is positioned front and centre of the UK's women's health strategy, and is a regular voice in national media, being frequently called upon to discuss topics concerning midlife and menopause.

Katie is the author of *The Not So Secret Diary of a Midlife Menopausal Mum* and *The Lockdown Diaries of a Midlife Menopausal Mum*. She lives in London with her husband and four children.

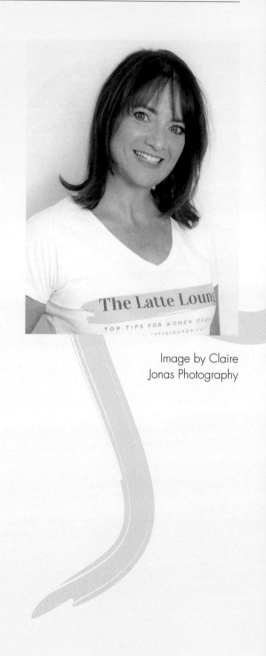

Image by Claire Jonas Photography

ACKNOWLEDGEMENTS

Thanks to my literary agent, Emily Sweet, for suggesting I write this book and for guiding me so patiently along the way. To the team at DK, I couldn't be happier or prouder of what we have created!

Thank you to my experts for all your contributions – whoever reads this book will have their lives changed for the better because of you. And, to the women who shared their experiences, thank you for trusting me to tell your stories.

Dedications

My husband Hugh: my rock, best friend, and cheerleader who has always believed in and loved me unconditionally. I'm so proud of everything you have achieved and grateful for all the fun and adventures we have been on together – here's to many more to come!

My children: Ellie, Josh, Sam, and Joe, my son-in-law Jake, and our cavachon Bobbie – thank you for bringing so much love, fun, turmoil, and entertainment. There's never a dull moment in our family and I wouldn't change it for the world. I love and am forever proud of you all.

Dad: thank you for passing down so many of the founding principles upon which I have built The Latte Lounge community: integrity, honesty, kindness,

compassion, a built-in "bullshit" radar, and a wicked sense of humour. I'm so proud of what you have achieved in your career as a breast cancer specialist – womankind owes you a huge debt of gratitude.

Mum: thank you for always quietly, modestly, and patiently supporting me through the good times and the bad. You have kept us all grounded and shown us how to live our lives to the full. I love and am very proud of you, too.

My siblings: Richard and Sue, I love you and your families very much and am super proud of your journalistic achievements.

The Taylors: marrying into the clan has totally enriched my life, bringing more warmth, fun, memories, and family than I could ever have wished for.

The Baums: I couldn't be prouder of all you've done for humankind: remarkable, considering our grandparents came to the UK as immigrants – Grandma Mary and Grandpa Isidor would be very proud.

My bestie Tor and all my friends, love you. Janice – you are forever missed.

My fellow MenoWarriors: never forget the difference us grassroots campaigners have made. We've moved mountains.

My Latte Lounge community and team (past and present): thank you for all your support; I'm incredibly proud of all that we have achieved together.

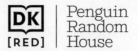

Senior Acquisitions Editor Zara Anvari
Editor Jasmin Lennie
Project Art Editor Jordan Lambley
Senior Production Controller Luca Bazzoli
Senior Production Editor Tony Phipps
Jacket Designer Jordan Lambley
Art Director Maxine Pedliham

Editorial Gaynor Sermon
Design Studio Noel
Illustration Charlotte Trounce

First published in Great Britain in 2025 by
DK RED, an imprint of
Dorling Kindersley Limited
20 Vauxhall Bridge Road,
London SW1V 2SA

The authorized representative in the EEA is
Dorling Kindersley Verlag GmbH. Arnulfstr.
124, 80636 Munich, Germany

A CIP catalogue record for this book
is available from the British Library.
ISBN: 978-0-2416-7445-1
Printed and bound in China

www.dk.com

PUBLISHER'S ACKNOWLEDGEMENTS

DK would like to thank all of the experts
involved for their insightful contributions,
Gaynor Sermon for piecing these together,
Studio Polka for the design concept, Kathy
Steer for proofreading, and Hilary Bird
for indexing.

DISCLAIMER

Neither the publisher nor the author
is engaged in rendering professional
advice or services to the individual reader.
The ideas, procedures, and suggestions
contained in this book are not intended
as a substitute for consulting with your
doctor or a professional. All matters
regarding your health require supervision.
Neither the author nor the publisher shall
be liable or responsible for any loss
or damage allegedly arising from any
information or suggestion in this book.

A NOTE ON GENDER IDENTITIES

DK recognizes all gender identities, and
acknowledges that the sex someone was
assigned at birth based on their sexual
organs may not align with their own
gender identity. People may self-identify
as any gender or no gender (including,
but not limited to, that of a cis or trans
woman, of a cis and trans man, or of a
non-binary person). As gender language,
and its use in our society evolves, scientific
and medical communities continue to
reassess their own phrasing. Most of
the studies referred to in this book use
"women" to describe people whose sex
was assigned as female at birth and "men"
to describe people whose sex was
assigned as male at birth.

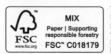